INVISIBLE
Battleground and The Non-Human Influence

Charles E. Nielsen

Copyright © 2024 by Charles E. Nielsen
All rights reserved.

Contents

Preface v
Chapter 1. 1
Chapter 2. 15
Chapter 3 25
Chapter 4 34
Chapter 5 38
Chapter 6 44
Chapter 7 48
Chapter 8 54
Chapter 9 63
Chapter 10 81
Chapter 11 92
Chapter 12 102
Chapter 13 108
Chapter 14 122
Chapter 15 131
Chapter 16 140
Chapter 17 146
Chapter 18 152
Chapter 19 162
Chapter 20 168
Epilogue 175

Preface

I wrote this book simply because I felt compelled to share what I believe has historical precedence that not many are focusing on concerning the struggles America and humanity faces in our world today.

This historical precedence that I'm referring to is often over looked and for many, simply not believed in.

Our world and our way of life seems to be coming apart at the seams and the traditional value systems are being attack, at every level.

Whether you're a person of faith or not, I hope that you'll take the time to read this book because there may be something you recognize as being valid in what is shared.

Most everything I address in this book is to relate that mankind, in one way or another, is being influenced by something we often can't see and is reflected in our policies.

I have not added a page of reference notes simply because most everything that I refer too in order to share with the reader has the access information or whom it was, on that page.

Everything and everyone I list has been out in the public but generally not on the mainstream news or publications platforms.

The mainstream news media and their social platforms have themselves become a source of misinformation and disinformation, yet accusing alternative platforms, that often times reveals the truth, of the very things they are doing.

In the end all of us must desire truth over what makes us feel good or what we want to believe.

If we can't do that, then we leave ourselves open for deception. We must try and find ways to avoid conflict, if at all possible, because the forces at work within our nation are hoping for a civil war to erupt in order to divide this nation.

It isn't just our nation that is facing troublesome times, it's the entire world at large.

Whether people believe it or not, we are not just in a physical struggle, we are in a spiritual struggle.

Many have no idea what it really means when I say we are in a spiritual struggle. My hope for those who have faith, will understand more clearly what that means and the dangers we face for the entire world.

Invisible Battleground and The Non-Human Influence

There are forces at work that are often never identified or even believed in. It's the cloak of disbelief that allows the deception to continue and once you recognize this unseen influence, you'll become more aware of the tactics that are being used to divide and then control.

Many have said what we are facing is from a small group of elites at the top that are the motivating force behind our turmoil today.

That would only be partly true. These elites are the second tier of influence, there is one above them.

We are at a cross-road and we're either going to stand together or fall prey to the invisible invading enemy that uses mankind like chest pieces.

Over the years there have been rumors of false flag events from outer-space. The UFO side has always been something that many elites believe would unite the world under a one world government if there were a threat from aliens from outer space. This idea started back around 1917.

However, the tables have been turned because the false flag event, was never going to be like the Independence Day attack like we see in the movie.

The attack started with the creation of mankind.

Chapter 1.

"In the end, there is a non-human connection to this global cult, this cult is a network, ultimately it is controlled by a non-human force ... manipulating society on behalf of a non-human force"
-David Ike - June 20, 2022

Book of Enoch - Chapter 19: *"Spirits assuming many different forms are defiling mankind and shall lead them astray."*

The Bible – Eph,9 6:12
12 For we are not fighting against flesh-and-blood enemies, but against evil rulers and authorities of the <u>unseen world</u>, against mighty powers in this dark world, and against evil spirits in the heavenly places.

David Ike

David Ike is a controversial figure that many may not give any validation. However, even controversial figures can get things right from time to time.

When David Ike mentions this global cult, he's referring to the elite that exist within organizations, institutions and governments that have the power to move and direct social and economic structure within countries and nations.

Groups such as the WEF (World Economic Forum) the WHO (World Health Organization) and the United Nations. It is a trinity of earthly power and control.

This includes very powerful yet unfamiliar names such as the Osini family whom, Pepe Orsini, is one of the most powerful with the connection of the Roman Papal Bloodline of the ancient Maximus family.

Magnus Maximus - World History Encyclopedia

Many researchers consider Pepe Osini the Gray Pope.

The Gray Pope is said to manage both the White Pope and the Black Pope and is believed to be the supreme ruler over of the entire world.

This is information that you will never hear over the mainstream news platforms.

Pepe Osini is believed to be a part of the secret and hidden thirteen Saturnalian Brotherhood of the Zoroastrian families who preside over the known thirteen illuminati families.

Pepe Orsini's linage can be traced back to 998AD and is known to be a major depopulationist, like most global elites. If Pepe Orsini is the grey Pope, then it is believed he is working along with the Black Pope in their Society of Jesus, otherwise known as the "Jesuits."

Jesuits, or Jesuit trained individuals, are known to have infiltrated or have been imbedded within all these highly powerful and influential organizations.

<u>Orsini Family | Italian Aristocrats & Papal Supporters | Britannica</u>

From these organizations are the tentacles that reach out to influence political operatives within the nations of the world that help shape global events. Events such as the Global "Great Reset.

Klaus Schwab founder of the WEF believes there must be a change in our world structure. Just what is that change they are seeking to establish?

Hillsdale College digest of liberty—author Michael Rectenwald described the economic goal of the Great Reset as "'capitalism with Chinese characteristics'—a two-tiered economy, with profitable monopolies and the state on top and socialism for the majority below."

On one hand it's to make changes to where people will except by free-will their proposals to restructure our existing world, and if not by free-will, through coercion.

That change is to bring about global control and to establish what many call a one world government. This change is now in progress and is taking place without much resistance. However, people are waking up!

Often times you need a catalyst or a primer that sets the wheels of change in motion. Like a war or a "pandemic."

This global reset was launched in 2019. A very convenient time. The planning has been in the works for decades with steps of strategically and incremental moves to bring about a step by step thorough global launch. It is called the "Great Reset Initiative." Klaus Schwab describes three points of this initiative:

1. Creating conditions for a "stakeholder economy." Stakeholders is a partnership of government and the private sector or corporations. More than likely, a part of that two-tiered system. I do believe the 'stakeholders' will be those at the very top of the food chain, not the average person on the street or those living under the socialist system.
2. Building in a more "resilient, equitable, and sustainable" way utilizing environmental, social and governance metrics (ESG). This is in line with what many call the Green New Deal. These are terms to increase greater central governmental control.
3. Harnessing the innovations of the "Fourth Industrial Revolution."

These points seem benign on the surface, even benevolent, but are they?

Some call the "Fourth Industrial Revolution" Industry 4.0, which is the rapid change to technology. This would include the rapid change in bio-technology and genetic alterations of mankind which involves quantum computing technology.

Within those three points are the matrix that promotes an organizational structure which will establish a campaign of propaganda and control over the entire world.

For the average person whom has little time to look into these set goals by the WEF, hear it and think, well they have our best interest in mind. They want to make things better for all of us; and it will sound that way too many of the uninformed.

The unfortunate truth is, NO, they don't have our best interest in mind. Not if you're a person who believes in liberty, personal responsibility and private property, those freedoms will need to be eliminated.

They don't openly come right out and say you'll lose your freedoms. They do come out and say at some point, you'll own nothing at all.

Their goal to control the world must be in language that will sound palatable and reasonable in order to combat any push back from those who catch on to their plan.

However, they will make the loss of those freedoms sound very reasonable and even logical. While many will go along with their plan, out of a lack of understanding what is taking place, others will go along in agreement.

Freedoms will need to be eliminated in a way that makes you feel-good about them being eliminated. You may not even realize they are eliminating your freedoms by the very words they use. They are very shrewd and use language and phycology that will appeal to the listener.

David Ike is spot on when he says society is being manipulated on behalf of non-human entities. It is about control and a new World Order.

If this is true then what is that non-human influence?

It is still hard for people to wrap their minds around the idea that there could be some invisible force or entity that could be influencing man-kind to take the direction we are heading in.

The idea of man being influenced by unseen forces isn't new, but in this modern age it appears to have been ignored or forgotten.

Book of Enoch

When the Book of Enoch mentions spirits taking many different "forms," it means mankind is being misled or deceived and influenced by unseen spirits or unseen entities. Influencing in many different ways. Ways that are often inconceivable to the rational mind.

These spirit that Enoch is talking about mentions the many different forms the unseen spirits take. As a noun, that covers many different manifestations, which include the physical to the spiritual. These spiritual entities can and do influence mankind on a conscientious level as well as the unconscientious mind.

If you come from a religious background or have a religious faith, then it's not beyond the reach to believe that there might be some kind of invisible influence of mankind. This invisible influence, whether good or bad, often starts in the mind of individuals.

Are all thoughts and ideas solely our own?

When Enoch talks about mankind being led astray, it can be an influence of wrong perceptions and thoughts from these unseen entities.

Let me give you one analogy of influencing spirits or entities. While this analogy is taken from a fictional program, it illustrates the effectiveness of these unseen influences that many people don't even believe is real.

The original Star Trek TV show was back in 1968. There was an episode where this invisible entity had infiltrated the Star Ship Enterprise. What the entity thrived and grew strong on was negative emotion, conflict and anger of individuals.

While the average viewer looked at this episode as sheer entertainment, the nuances of the show revealed something quite interesting.

It revealed that the entity was able to get people, who would normally view a situation rationally with logic, to now see things irrational and to make them believe they were thinking, rational.

The unseen entity induced suspicion, anger and rage, in situations that would normally or rationally not be present.

Could invisible forces be affecting our society today?

You may have heard the saying, they had a monkey on their back. It's an idiom reference to what someone may be struggling with in their life. It can be a metaphor to something unseen effecting a person; referring to an issue that is troubling people physically or emotionally.

Everyone, no matter who they are, will struggle with an issue or weakness in their life. We all have areas of weakness in our lives. Sometimes those issues or weaknesses are hidden from the public and kept in the dark regions of our minds. Other times they consume a person's life to the point where they struggle daily to even function. That is one battleground and there "may or may not be" an invisible influence to that struggle. It can originate from our past experiences that affect us psychologically but also spiritually.

However, there are influencing spirits that can cause turmoil in our life and in our society. Often times we don't look at it as an influencing spirit, just bad judgement; and sometimes, that's all it is. Other times it is an unidentified or unacknowledged adversarial spirit.

The further we get away from our spiritual foundation, the less capable we are to recognize the influence.

The Invisible Battleground and Non-Human Influence I'm referring too isn't just depression or despair coming from a chemical imbalance, abuse or even addiction that inhibits an individual's life on a daily basis or some unfortunate circumstance.

The invisible battle that I'm referring to is that struggle that takes place in the unseen realm that mankind faces. It is the spiritual battle that affect mankind collectively and on a global scale. This battle is taking place right now on the world stage.

Eph 6:12

There is an invisible (evil) influence that affects the elite and leaders of our world; of how they think and the direction they take. They can appear as men and women of righteous character, and yet be ravenous wolves behind the scenes.

Let me paint a picture for you. This struggle is about good vs evil.

The typical view of good vs evil we see today is a picture of a person on the right, many portray as Jesus as the good. Then a person on the left that appears to be the typical picture of the devil in red with a pitch fork, horns and a tail, as evil.

While that has been our typical picture of the struggle of good vs evil. Evil can be overt or covert. Evil can appear as an angel of light or even something good.

2 Cor 11:14

14 "And no wonder, for even Satan disguises himself as an angel of light." ESV

The Bible writer of Ephesians 6:12 points out that there is an invisible realm that has a power structure and that mankind's battle is not necessarily just physical but fought in the unseen world.

The battleground I'm referring too here is the invisible influences that most people don't even realize are there and yet has been there from the beginning of mankind. It's the kind of invisible-battle that affect us through our institutions and the governments of the world.

It is an invisible evil force, unseen, unknown and unacknowledged by most today. This unseen force (which is the non-human influence) can manipulate the thinking pattern on an individual level or in the high rankings of world governments and has its impact throughout history.

The bible writer warned of an adversary that uses our mind. Almost like that Star Trek episode where the invisible force attacked their thinking process.

2 Cor 2:*11* ***"that no advantage may be gained over us by Satan: for we are not ignorant of his devices."*** ASV

This word "devices" in the Greek is "noee'mata or "noema" and means our own minds. That is the device this unseen force can use.

This unseen force often times influences the leaders of this world and those elites that seem to pull the strings of governments. Of course fear, depression and despair can be a tool to be used by this unseen force, not just on individuals but collectively. Often time's government is the active arm of this unseen force, because it is not only invisible, it is generally not even believed in.

This invisible influence helps shape the mind of man and the events in our world today, as it has from the beginning.

Take for example, Adam and Eve in the garden of Eden. Some may consider it an allegory. No matter how you look at the story, whether literal or allegorical, it is the outside influence (the serpent) upon Eve that swayed her to choose a direction to disobeyed God, the creator.

For the sake of our discussion, we'll call the serpent a dimensional or divine being.

Also a note of interest, when it refers to the "serpent" in Hebrews, it is actually referring to an Elohim or divine being that Jehovah created.

Gen 3:1-6

"The serpent was the shrewdest the Lord God had made. One day he asked the woman, "Did God really say you must not eat the fruit from any of the trees in the garden?"

2 "Of course we may eat fruit from the trees in the garden," the woman replied. 3 "It's only the fruit from the tree in the middle of the garden that we are not allowed to eat. God said, 'You must not eat it or even touch it; if you do, you will die.'"

4 "You won't die!" the serpent replied to the woman. 5 "God knows that your eyes will be opened as soon as you eat it, and you will be like God, knowing both good and evil." 6 The woman was convinced."

This adversary knows the psychology of the human mind and uses it against mankind.

I suspect that Eve was presented to disobey God in a way that looked like the right thing to do at that time or that she could be like her creator; even looking at it in a way that she may have thought, this was a test to become more knowledgeable. If not a test, a temptation to be like her creator.

Bad or misleading influences can look attractive, tempting or even the right thing to do. When we feel the temptation, often times when we know it's not the right thing to do, we find ways to justify it in our minds to make it appear right or acceptable, especially if it's appealing to us.

Not to get off track here but it's almost like raising children.

When raising children we watch over them and do our best to make sure they don't come into contact with wrong influences. We guard or protect over those bad influences that are seen. But what about unseen influences they come in contact with and seem to change the very demeanor of the child?

It is the unseen influences upon our mind and how we look at situations that can be misleading. This very approach happens in our world leaders to sway them and to gain power that is often times deleterious to the population and at the same time, these leaders who are motivated by their hunger for power and by an unseen influence, make bad policies and rules that appear appealing to the people, (shrewd and deceptive).

These policies of government, influenced by non-human entities, may sound and look positive on the surface, are the instruments of the pied piper. In other words, deceiving the public with very appealing and attractive promises to gain greater control by the government.

Battle of the Mind

Professions of psychiatry and psychology over the years has been a great help to many who are struggling in their life. On occasion when improper or unprincipled methods and techniques are used, great harm and more confusion to those struggling are the results.

In their profession, their goal is to help understand the mind and how it copes with issues that we often face. At one point in my life I myself wanted to go into the field of psychology because I found it interesting on how people think and perceive – I'm thankful I didn't.

I spent years in the study of Bible-scripture and history. The old saying is, the more you learn the more you realize how little you know, stands true.

However in my studies over the years I've not only read about this unseen influence, but come to recognize that this unseen influence cannot only influence people individually, it's actually manipulating world leaders in a direction that laid the course of humanity; not only in the past but also our present day and for the future. However only up to a point.

Chapter 2.

Where Does This Unseen Influence Come From and Who or What Might It Be?

Have you ever been away from city lights at night and just looked up into the sky and seen all the stars and even the Milky Way and think, wow - how amazing! How did we come to exist? Is there other life out there?

Most people of faith have a belief in the spiritual dimension. They believe there is a creator of mankind. Every religion has a creation story. Often times that belief in the spiritual dimension very seldom attributes any kind of influence to world leaders. It's usually on individuals who are affected by a positive or negative spirit or what some may call demons.

Yet throughout history we see written records about the gods of the past that have influenced the kings and kingdoms of this world; yet today we seem to be completely silent on that outside or unseen influence.

Heather Lynn, PhD wrote the book Evil Archaeology. I don't believe she is a Christian or coming from a Christian point of view in her book.

However it appears that she does believe in a spiritual evil influence that has been recorded throughout history.

The spirit world is the dimensional world these entities exist in and influence nations.

From the *How&Why's* article by Vicky Verma 9/9/23, "George Knapp of Coast to Coast late night radio talk show said, he knows someone high-ranking who told him that human conflict, specifically war, is sometimes intentionally designed by a malevolent non-human intelligence through manipulation."

He's talking about entities that are possibly dimensional and somehow manipulating mankind through the mind. The religious world has seen them as evil spirits.

History is replete with accounts of the unseen influence governments had.

Adolf Hitler: Obsessed with the Occult (historynet.com) Eric Kurlander points out about Germany in the late 1930s that Dr. Bernard Hormann headed up a pro-enlightenment effort. The Nazis felt that there was great deceptions among the so-called "un-educated or un-enlightened." They believed in the occult spirit world.

Joseph Goebbels the Nazi propagandist encouraged a scientific look into astrology. They used astrology as a tool that influenced their direction of invasions and counter intelligence.

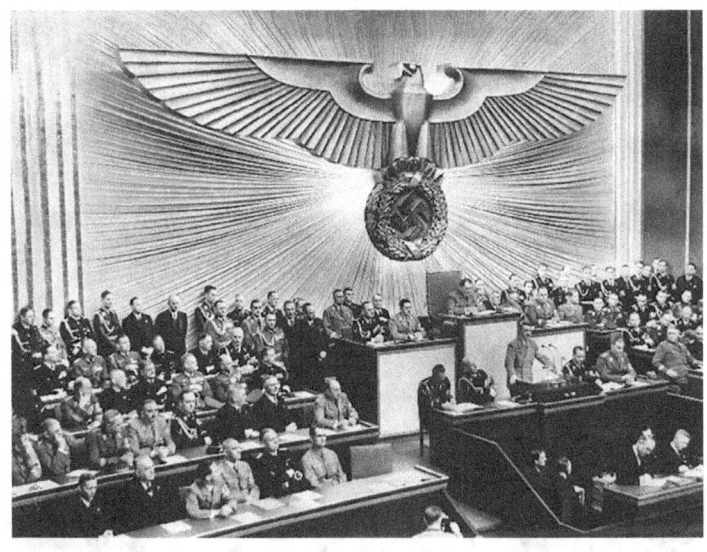

Since that time, science has worked hard to eliminate the spiritual from their equations. Meaning, you're irrational if you believe in the spiritual or even the paranormal as to influencing leaders of the world today.

Yet part of the U.S. government did believe in what some called fringe science of remote viewing with the Star Gate project.

Even though part of our government used paranormal science behind the eyes of the public, with the help of our educational system we no longer believe in the spiritual side or the mythological gods because we consider ourselves more advanced; at least the public at large no longer believes in them.

There just the beliefs of primitive ancient people of the past. We're more sophisticated today and don't believe in all the silly mythological gods or the paranormal. Yet the elite of our world today may have a different position on that.

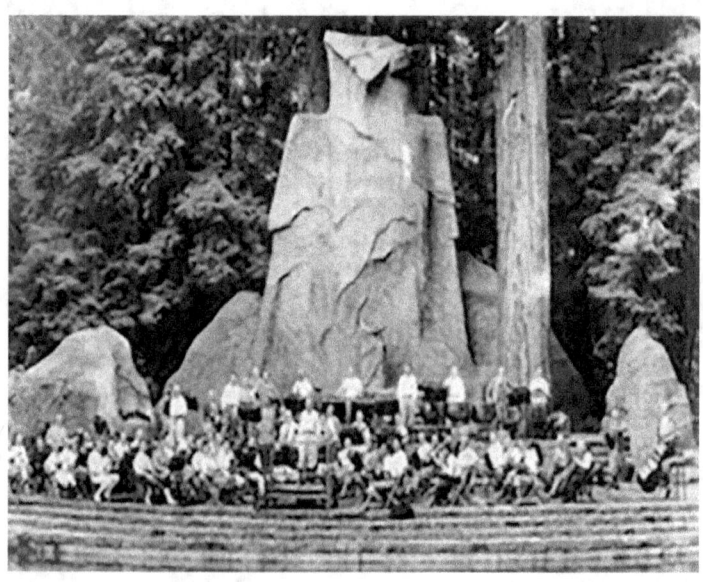

Regardless of what you may think about Alex Jones, the man who is the face of "Info-Wars." He was the only one who was able to infiltrate the secretive meetings at the Bohemian Grove in California where influential people and world leaders meet and preform mock sacrifices to a forty foot Owl god (Moloch). Why? Why would they do that?

We are talking about presumed sophisticated leaders of the world today who believe in acting out a mock sacrifice to a pagan god. To many of us that's a bazaar act.

Yet this all has a spiritual influence behind their actions.

From Rense.com The Significance Of Bohemian Grove Owl Worship (rense.com)

The article points this out:

"Owl medicine is symbolically associated with clairvoyance, astral projection, and magic, both black and white. Owl's called the Night Eagle on several medicine wheels used by Amerindian teachers. Traditionally, Owl sits in the East, the place of illumination (as many Masonic Temples point East). Since time immemorial, humanity has been afraid of the night, the dark, and the unseen – waiting fearfully for the first crack of morning light. Conversely, night is Owl's friend. . .

Owl medicine is a form of worship.

You'll see from Joe Rogan YouTube clip of Alex Jones laying out the history of the Bohemian Grove and describes the evil that exists in this circle of people. You can even validate it for yourself.

(30) Alex Jones on Bohemian Grove, Skull & Bones, Epstein – YouTube

With all of the evil that is taking place in our world today, we have to ask; could it be the influence of those same entities of the past that God himself reprimanded for allowing evil and are now influencing the leaders of modern times?

Ps 82:1-2

*"**God has taken his place in the divine council;
in the midst of the <u>gods</u> he holds judgment:
2 "How long will you judge unjustly
and show partiality to the wicked?"*** ESV

Ps 82 is talking about the creator of all things (John 1:1-3) who created these other gods, who were once a part of his council and then rebelled. They established all these other religions and cultures of the world. He is reprimanding them for allowing evil and partiality to the wicked.

Who were these gods that Jehovah was reprimanding?

These gods of the past run into the thousands and the many religions of our world. You had the gods of:

- Greeks
- Egyptians
- Norse
- Romans
- Hindu

- Aztec
- Celtic
- Japanese
- Mayan
- Chinese
- Babylonian

There are many more than listed here.

You had lessor entities posing as gods of weather, peace and even war; such as the god of war, *Kukailimoku* who was the family god of the chieftain Kamehameha from the Hawaiian Islands

<u>List of Gods and Goddesses From Antiquity (learnreligions.com)</u>

<u>Those same entities that Jehovah God was reprimanding are the same invisible entities that are influencing our world leaders and those in powerful positions today, and a dark part of our government knows this.</u>

The History Channel did a segment on the Bohemian Grove and concluded that nothing "nefarious" was taking place there; at least what they were allowed to see.

Coming from a Christian perspective I would have to disagree. I also believe had they truly found or mentioned something of a nefarious nature to the secular world, it would have never made it to the screen of the History Channel.

Even the History Channel representative said they do believed that if something nefarious was taking place (or revealed) it probably wouldn't have remained on the YouTube channel since YouTube fact-checkers remove anything they may disagree with.

That position due to what YouTube fact-checker believe is acceptable, may also be nefarious to the Christian position.

Influencing spirits can often be found in secret societies and especially within the elites.

(30) Brad Meltzer's Decoded: Secret Societies Uncovered (S1, E9) | Full Episode | History – YouTube

President John F. Kennedy on April 27th 1961 at the Waldorf-Astoria Hotel, New York said: "The very word secrecy is repugnant in a free and open society, and we as a people inherently and historically, opposed to secret societies, to secret oaths and secret proceedings."

This is exactly what is taking place among world leaders and the very powerful. Many of these world leaders may have no idea or even believe they are being influenced by the unseen non-human entities; and yet, some may knowingly be seeking the unseen for direction.

Now for those that do not believe in the spiritual side. This is nonsense to them. I understand that. And there is not much one can do to convince a person that holds that position.

It is true, people will believe what they want to believe, rather than what might be true. It's about a piece of reluctance in all of us to accept or believe something that we initially didn't believe in or thought was not possible…to what degree that keeps us from accepting the truth revealed by historical data and scripture? It depend on whether a person is open enough to allow truth that will supersede their hurt feelings.

To truly understand what is taking place in the Invisible Battleground, means you cannot be an unbeliever in the spiritual things and identify this unseen force. <u>You virtually blind yourself by your unbelief.</u>

1 Cor 2:14

*14 **Now the natural man does not receive the things of the Spirit of God: for they are foolishness unto him; and he cannot know them, because they are spiritually judged.*** (Spiritually understood)

This unbelief is in part what these entities rely upon. It is the cloak of disbelief that allows them to continue to shape world events through their surrogates.

These entities who influence our world are the beings that Jehovah created and then rebelled. They also display or reveal themselves in many different forms: UFOs, ghosts, poltergeists, spirits of past loved ones, cryptic creatures, through crop circles and many different species of aliens, etc. This is where Enoch points out that these spirits defile mankind and take many different forms in order to lead them away from the truth.

When we talk about angels or fallen angels, we are referring to a job title and they can appear as an angel of light.

2 Cor 11:14

The Hollywood version of Satan is pitchfork and horns. The reality is, he and his worker can portray themselves as something good and beneficial to mankind.

We have been conditioned over the years that the spiritual enemy of mankind must look and sound a certain way for us to recognize evil. That isn't how it works. Deception works on many different levels, some open and blatant. Others can look and be beneficial at the beginning and have long term repercussions.

Often times leading mankind in the wrong direction is not done by huge leaps but rather small incremental moves. There is another term that conveys the same sentiment. Death by a ten-thousand tiny cuts.

Chapter 3

Invisible Influence of Demoralization and Loss of Virtue How America Lost its way

You've probably heard over the last few years people say something to the effect, 'what has happened to our world? Things seem to be upside down.'

The reason for some of those comments is due to what used to be considered common-sense in our society, has now become uncommon or not in the range of practical or rational.

In other words and on some topics or issues, right has become wrong and wrong has become right. Traditional virtue and logic has given way to a new paradigm.

It is the goal of influencing spirits to disrupt and to change the norms of society. In doing so brings about confusion and a demoralization, devaluation and loss of virtue is their goal.

June 19th 2023 the headline from the Blaze read: **"Student excoriated, called "Homophobic" for**

refusing to accept that her classmate identifies as a cat."

Also June 19th 2023 from the Blaze: **"Book bans' are castrating children: Maryland Gov. Wes Moore demands 'economic consequences' for states removing sexually explicit books from schools"**

Who in their right mind would want to keep porn in the schools?

Again from Blaze News Headlines, (which covers news that the mainstream refuse to cover) Sept. 1, 2023, **"Oklahoma DRAG QUEEN hired as elementary school principle despite former child pornography charges."**

Also **"Gender Hybrids" – Professor Claims Children Identify as 'MINOTAURS' Are Leading the Gender Revolution"** Story by S. Salmaan 2023.

Even some who consider themselves liberal, believe this has gone too far.

It appears that irrational positions on a number of issues have been considered, rational in our world today.

How many times have you heard some leader, either in government, in a movement or an organization, say something that is irrational, and try to make it sound as though it is rational and normal? Then say to yourself, that doesn't sound right or rational! Or that doesn't make any sense! Yet the people taking ill-rational positions believe its right or at least they try and convince you it's right, when you know it's wrong.

It's about the loss of virtue. Virtue helps in the development of positive and rational thinking and decision making. Virtue was credited with the rise of Rome, but then the loss off virtue was credited with the fall of Rome.

Virtue provides: Liberty (meaning our freedom and personal responsibility), morality, prosperity and the security of a nation. The lack of virtue will produce a perversion of "meaning and logic" and affect every aspect of our lives. This is why many of us recognize, right has become wrong and wrong has become right.

As an example. The FAA will seek to hire people with severe disabilities. From their web site: "They include hearing, vision, missing extremities, partial paralysis, complete paralysis, epilepsy, severe intellectual disability, psychiatric disability and dwarfism."

Jan. 15th 2024

FAA seeks to hire people with 'severe intellectual' and 'psychiatric' problems in DEI push – what could go wrong? (bizpacreview.com)

It's a spiritual war being played out in our corporal world. In other words, those who are influenced by the wrong spirit manifests itself in our physical world or in their actions. This has been a historical warning from the scriptures to all of us about a breakdown of society, rational thinking, a demoralization and why it happens.

A "demoralization" means: to throw a person into disorder, confusion and bewilderment. That is exactly what many recognize today taking place within our nation and culture. Virtue, honesty and decency have almost become a "pariah."

Isa 5:20-21:

***What sorrow for those who say
that evil is good and good is evil,
that dark is light and light is dark,
that bitter is sweet and sweet is bitter.
21 What sorrow for those who are wise in their own eyes
and think themselves so clever.***

This has happened throughout history and scripture reveals that when man starts to remove himself from virtue *(quality of high moral standards)* his world view goes from a rational to irrational and of right and wrong to where wrong looks right and right looks wrong.

It happens slowly and incrementally that sucks society and cultures along its destructive path.

We often look at the Roman Empire as always being decadent and debased in its morals. However that isn't true. Rome actually gave credit to its rise in power due to their virtue and strong moral values.

Ancient Roman Moral Principles | Maria Milani Ancient Rome

> - The early Roman Empire gave credit to the rise of its empire from virtue. A value system early that started out in honesty and character. From Maria Milani site called, ***Ancient Rome Moral Principles:* "Virtues:**
> - Specific morals and virtues expected of individuals. Typical terms used were '**gravitas**', '**pietas**', '**dignitas**' for men and '**pudicitia**' for women. Gravitas was particularly of importance during the early part of the Roman Republic. The historian Polibius remarked on how the honesty and virtues and honesty of early Republican Roman officials was a marked advantage for the rise of Rome versus other cultures such as Greece.

It means Rome started out with a principle that is universally beneficial to all mankind, which is honesty and dignity (character). Those virtues were a foundation of both men and women and for a prosperous society. The word Pudicitia means modesty in women.

Much like our founding principles for America when two of our founders said:

"A free people cannot survive under a republican constitution unless they remain virtuous and morally strong. "Only a virtuous people are capable of freedom. As nations become corrupt and vicious, they have more need of masters." - Benjamin Franklin

"The most promising method of securing a virtuous people is to elect virtuous leaders. "Neither the wisest constitution nor the wisest laws will secure the liberty and happiness of a people whose manners are universally corrupt. He therefore is the truest friend to the liberty of his country who tries most to promote its virtue, and who ... will not suffer a man to be chosen into any office of power and trust who is not a wise and virtuous man." - Samuel Adams

We can see how America has followed in the very footsteps of the Roman Empire, from its beginning to the corruption we have today. Revelations 13:11-18. Maria Milani points out:

> By the time the threat was over to individuals' wellbeing and Julius Caesar had done his part to put an end to the Republic and open the way to a dictatorial Empire, "things", from a moral point of view, took a liberal turn for the next three or four centuries(2017),

This means, the Republican government of Rome was removed (no doubt without the people realizing it happened) which at the beginning had a foundation in virtue and leaders of high moral character, that gave to its rise, then moving into a liberalism of changing values along with a growing and more restrictive and invasive government.

We are repeating history because we've failed to look back at history and to avoid the pitfalls of a changing moral value system.

Milani points out:

> The sort of morality delivered from a pulpit often, if not always, made reference to the "good old" days when Romans, true Romans, led their austere life. Sticking to moralist tradition at the service of the greatness of Rome was vigorously upheld by the likes of Cato the Elder (234-149BC) and Emperor Augustus (2017).

It cannot be over stated here that the influence and temptation of moral permissiveness started the chain reaction to Rome's eventual down fall, *as* Milani points out in her further statement of Rome:

> It is at this point, when talking of the end of the empire, that it is useful to recall what was said at the very beginning of this article: that morality is a product of the people who live by it. It is therefore easy to consider that the fall of Roman society was not a sudden collapse caused by orgies, dissolution, corruption and the barbaric invasions of Rome!

> What we regularly observe nowadays was true then also: The society living in the provinces north and south of Rome required time to be <u>influenced</u> by what occurred in the capital (or Capitol!) As such the customs and solidity of society and indeed their customs and moral structure lived on in the provinces, even when the nerve center of Rome had long given way.
>
> The same is applicable to the reverse wave of morality brought by Christianity: Christianity eventually did away with the pagan view of society which had long been associated with a failing morality but it took some time before the effects of Christianity saw their way through to the provinces and indeed through to the rest of Europe (2017).

It can be said the same for America. America's fall in our moral foundation was not sudden but on a gradual decline to where we are today.

You can go back from where we are today to 40-50 years ago and you would never see: Drag Queen days in school, gender reassignment and counselling without the consent of the parents, even porn available to our children in their libraries; 40–50 years ago, anyone who would suggest those be a part of the school curriculum, would immediately be thrown out of their positions and considered perverse.

Change never happens overnight, especially if it's the type of change that is going against an established societal moral norms. Those types of changes are slow and incrementally.

However, some changes can happen fast given the right circumstances.

Chapter 4

Tools Used by Unseen Entities that shape society

Tools used by unseen entities are in fact mankind being played like chest pieces. Individuals, those in leadership are influenced in their thought processes to create rules and policies that can change the world. Once put into action can change things culturally and sometimes at a fast pace.

Journalist Katrina Trinko wrote an article in the Daily Signal March 27th 2023. In the article Trinko points out some very interesting developments as a results of the Covid19 plandemic. Yes I did say "Plandemic" because I do believe what took place with Covid19, was deliberate. My position is supported by a Chinese scientist defector.

While I can't put Katrina Trinko's entire article in my book due to not having permission; which was an excellent article. I will relay some of the poignant data she revealed.

As a results of the Covid19 pandemic there was a drastic change in our American values. It was a change that took a mere two to three years.

Katrina Trinko points out that in 2019 prior to the Covid19 pandemic a Wall Street Journal/NBC News poll showed that 89% of Americans believed hard work was very important. It also showed that 62% believed community involvement was vital. It showed that 6 out of 10 believed that patriotism was crucial. Nearly half Americans (48%) felt religion was important and at 43% believe having children was very important.

Then a new Wall Street Journal conducted by NORC at the University of Chicago found that all those values had dropped over a short period of time.

What took place was, Covid19 hit and shutdowns happened. People were laid off, many small business owners went out of business and we were told to shelter in place. They couldn't be out and about mingling and mixing with large groups of people. You couldn't congregate in Church. You were required to wear a mask in many department and food stores.

In Monterey and Carmel California they had signs up that stated, if you didn't wear a mask, there was a $100 fine. It was literally depriving people of their constitutional rights.

After a mere two to three years, a big change took place.

The new poll showed the belief in hard work as a value dropped from 89% to 67%. Patriotism dropped from basically 60% down to now 38%. The importance of religion and having children dropped from 48% and 43% to 39% and 30%. And as far as community involvement, that dropped from 62% down to a whopping, 25%.

What was the major factor in these changes? "Government promoted Fear through the health departments." Media and the government working in unison to promote greater government control over the people. While those at the very top knew they were lying to the public. But for what purpose?

As I have mentioned earlier in this book, government is often the arm/tool to be wheeled by outside and unseen influences. Mandates: of mask, vaccines, churches shut down, you couldn't congregate and you had to shelter in place and the removal of our constitutional rights. All of which were very unscientific but claiming they were supported by science.

In some places if you were on the streets you had to have papers showing you were a vital worker and it was necessary for you to be on the road or out in public.

These are the tools to help bring people under control and even to demoralize them.

While BLM (Black Lives Matters a Marxist group) and ANTIFA (A claimed anti-fascist group who are actually fascists) could riot burn down buildings and congregate in large crowds without any real penalties.

The very government that was supposed to protect the Constitution, the people's rights and freedoms, were now stripping those rights away, all under the false narrative that Covid19 would kill you if you didn't obey the government sponsored health officials and its lockdowns.

Chapter 5

Hidden in Plain Sight?

Is it possible that there are entities that we can't see somehow influencing our world today?

Helen Sharman, Britain's first astronaut and a chemist at Imperial College London, believes that alien lifeforms, that we cannot see or recognize, may be living among us.

[Could invisible aliens really exist among us? An astrobiologist explains (theconversation.com)](#)

What some may reveal might be on a microbial level but what about something more than just microbes?

David M. Jacobs, PhD and author of *Walking Among US* has spent decades into the investigation of people who claim they've been abducted by UFO's. Dr. Jacobs is an American historian and retired Associate Professor of History at Temple University specializing in 20th-century American history.

In his book and his interviews, Dr. Jacobs points out that what he came to believe was very hard for him to accept. He's not a conspiracy theorist. He didn't want to believe what his research was showing him but could no longer deny the data.

The very idea of extraterrestrial beings out there in the universe is believed by many in the science community. However, they believe that the reason we haven't made contact or found evidence of extraterrestrial life is simply because of the expanse of space (of course evidence has been all around us). For the mainstream scientists believe it's just too far for them to reach us. (I believe that position to be hubris).

And of course these same scientists completely ignore the possibility of a creator or God that has beings that may travel in a dimensional realm. Or colloquially speaking, who have the ability to pop in and out of our dimension.

Diana Brown's article from the website *How Stuff Works* points out about dimensions: ". . . for string theory to be accurate, (the theory that connects everything) it means there could be more than 10 dimensions, instead of the four we're used to experiencing: length, width, depth and time. Some of these dimensions could theoretically be places where the Big Bang never happened and the universe had an entirely different starting point. What would a creature from a dimension like that look like to humans from the fourth dimension? Lovecraftian monsters? Demogorgons?"

Are Creatures Living Among Us in Parallel Dimensions? | HowStuffWorks

The point I'm making here is, many highly educated people do believe there could be influences or things taking place around us that we simply cannot see and they may not have our best interest in mind. As Dr. David Jacobs believes that while he thought just maybe extraterrestrial beings were interested in us as a species, what he came to believe was just the opposite. He believes what is taking place is a planetary acquisition. That obviously isn't a good thing.

It is almost like the movie called *They Live* where the invading aliens were walking among the human population undetected. You needed special glasses to see them.

Dr. Jacobs knows how difficult it is for people to believe this and does not come from a religious or spiritual point of view. He simply comes from a data collection extrapolation. He knows how difficult it is for people to believe what he's saying. However, Dr. Jacobs has interviewed over 1,000 people and through hypnotherapy he has collected corroborating data that led him to his conclusion.

How Invisible Entities Influence the Mind

We may wonder, if there are invisible adversary's shaping world events and society, how are they doing it?

The invisible entities often use tactics of dividing: by economic class, race, religion, sexual identities, political identity, social customs, language or nationalities etc. They use the subconscious mind as the starting point of division.

As an illustration for unseen influence.

Years ago I came across an article about advertising in department stores. The article was referring to a law suit that was filed against one of the big department chain stores, claiming they were using subliminal messages within the music they were playing over the store.

They were making the claim that even though you couldn't outwardly hear the message, it was placed within the music so your mind would receive it without you realizing it, and hopefully compel you to buy more. The suit was claiming unethical practices by the department store.

Subliminal messages seem to work through sight and sound.

The word "subliminal" has an interesting definition from Merriam-Websters: "Since the Latin word *limen* means «threshold», something subliminal exists just below the threshold of conscious awareness. The classic example of a subliminal message is «Eat popcorn» flashed on a movie screen so quickly that the audience doesn›t even notice it consciously."

There has been a great deal of attention to the science of subliminal influence. Jonah Berger wrote the book called *Invisible Influence* where he says this:

"There's a funny story that I mention briefly in the book. A number of years ago, my dad was buying a new car. He lives in Washington, D.C. He's a lawyer there. He bought a BMW. Then he was complaining that all D.C. lawyers buy BMWs. I said, "Well, Dad, you bought a BMW also." He said, "Oh, but mine's a blue one. Everyone else drives a gray one."

For Jonah Berger's father it was the social influence of those in his profession that influenced him to buy a BMW. He justified his action as not following the crowd by him buying a blue one that made him feel as though he wasn't totally influenced.

Subliminal-advertising is that which contains: words, images, or sounds designed to convey a message to an audience that the conscious mind can't perceive. In other words, subliminal advertising uses visual and auditory stimuli to influence the subconscious mind and drive consumer behavior, while the consumer isn't consciously aware of the message that's being conveyed. The hope by the influencer is to drive greater product purchasing.

Whether it is a consumer based or socially based influence, we all face it and sometime succumb to it.

If it's socially based influence, it can, at times, be called mob mentality. Everyone seems to be doing this or having that and compels us to justify the same action.

Sometimes the collective action or social influence is benign and may have no detrimental effect on society.

However, let's say the government uses the tool of fear to motivate the citizenry; it can affect the very freedoms and rights of its citizens. Given the right circumstance it can actually make citizens turn on each other; not realizing that the influence to take that action against its own citizens, was motivated by fear or hate and promoted by the government.

We see the evidence of what took place to the Jews in Germany when the government promoted fear and hate against the Jewish people in the late 1930s and early 1940s.

Our government through the arm of mainstream media and social platforms promoted fear against those who refused to take the Covid19 vaccine or refused to wear a mask that never did work.

Many in the medical field who were silenced by the government, claimed what took place for Covid19, masks and vaccines, was a mass-formation-psychosis, or in other words, a mass-brainwashing by our government sponsored health department. Many today are still under the spell of our government's sorcery and believe everything the government tells them.

It was literally turning citizen against citizen.

Chapter 6

Entities that Use Subconscious and Dream Influence

It's important to understand that many of the great men and women felt they had outside influences that helped them. From: Pythagoras to Einstein, Tesla and many others believed they were influenced outside of human contact.

> The spiritual side that influences mankind may take place while we are awake or asleep.

Within the spiritual realm, influence can also come through dreams. In the Old Testament Job gives the account of how God works telling people that God does communicate but people just don't always recognize it.

I'm using the Living Translation so the language can be better understood:

Job 33:12-15

**"But you are wrong, and I will show you why.
For God is greater than any human being.
13 So why are you bringing a charge against him?
Why say he does not respond to people's complaints?
14 For God speaks again and again,
though people do not recognize it.
15 He speaks in dreams, in visions of the night,
when deep sleep falls on people
as they lie in their beds."**

You may have read where I have mentioned that Jehovah God created the beings that brought about all the religions of this world. These beings (again, some call aliens others call fallen angels) function on a vibrational and consciousness level. As Jehovah God does, they too (adversarial spirits) can enter a person's dreams, placing thoughts, ideas and visions.

As an example. The Indian mathematician **Srinivasa Ramanujan**, (born December 22, 1887 was one of the greatest mathematicians in history. Still influencing us today with his mathematical theorems.

Srinivasa Ramanujan was obsessed with mathematics. He dropped out of high school and continued to work on his math. He worked night and day and came up with hundreds of different ways of calculating approximate values of pi. In just two notebooks he wrote around 400 pages of formulas and theorems. Thanks to his work the theoretical foundations that Ramanujan gave us over a century ago, have helped powerful computers calculate the first 10 trillion decimals of the number pi.

Srinivasa Ramanujan claimed that it was the goddess, Namagiri, who showed him in dreams the equations of his formulas.

[Ramanujan, the Man who Saw the Number Pi in Dreams | OpenMind (bbvaopenmind.com)](#)

The very realm of the unseen is where these divine beings exist and operate. Scripture reveals that whether a person believes they are alien or fallen angels, it was God through Christ who created these dimensions and powers.

Col 1:15

**"for through him God created everything
in the heavenly realms and on earth.
He made the things we can see
and the things we can't see—
such as thrones, kingdoms, rulers, and authorities in
the unseen world." LNT.**

There is a power structure within the fallen angel realm that created the religions of this world.

Even now those in our government and former government officials are saying that non-human beings are here and may be functioning on a conscientious and vibrational level.

The mainstream press will never report on what is being revealed.

Those who are not afraid to share the truth will be detached from the corporate controlled media that is now starting to produce Artificial Intelligent delivered news.

An article by Vicky Verma written on 9/9/2023 Titled *'Extraterrestrials See Humans as 'Containers of Souls'* point out that alien beings "thrive" on lower vibrational energy and emotions such as; fear, anger, hate, depression etc. Very much like the Star Trek show I mentioned earlier.

What is coming to light is the fact that our government knows about this, as bazaar as this may sound. Some of this information is now starting to leak out through the government whistle-blower program.

Chapter 7

Government Whistle Blower

You may be wondering, what does government whistle blowers have to do with the non-human influence this book is talking about?

This gives us a picture of entities that are often unseen and yet can take physical form that our government, not only knows about, but has kept hidden from the public for decades.

David Charles Grusch, is a U.S. Air Force veteran at the rank of Major and was an intelligence official. Grusch is also "a decorated former combat officer in Afghanistan, and a veteran of the National Geospatial-Intelligence Agency (NGA) and the National Reconnaissance Office (NRO). He served as the reconnaissance office's representative to the Unidentified Aerial Phenomena Task Force from 2019-2021. From late 2021 to July 2022, he was the NGA's co-lead for UAP analysis and its representative to the task force.

David Charles Grusch is now a UFO/UAP whistleblower who claims the government is in possessing of what he calls "intact and partially intact craft of non-human origin." This according to The Debrief article and reaffirmed at the congressional hearings on UFO/UAPs.

The Debrief first broke the story about Grusch's accusations on June 5, 2023. Grusch later spoke with NewsNation and repeated the claims at the congressional hearings.

The reason he broke the story with the Debrief was because he felt in danger from our government and felt his life was in danger.

According to the Debrief Grusch has given Congress and the Intelligence Community Inspector General extensive classified information about a deeply covert programs" involving the alleged alien aircraft.

The Inspector General called this claim urgent and credible. The reason the Inspector General called it urgent and credible is because of who David Grusch is. He is one of the most credible whistle blowers in recent history to come forward with his claims.

David Grusch claims that part of the government that has been involved with the UFO/UAPs have kept this all away from congress and the public.

David Grusch believes the government (or a part of the government) has been illegally holding these alien crafts in their possession.

David Grusch filed a complaint alleging that he suffered retaliation. He said that it has been a nightmare experience for him and for his confidential disclosure. He believes what our government is doing to be illegal.

The outlet also reported that it has obtained similar, corroborating information from other intelligence officials, both active and retired, with knowledge of these programs. They believe David Grusch is legitimate and credible.

It's important to note that Grusch has credible support: Retired Army Colonel Karl E. Nell, who worked with Grusch on the UAP Task Force, shared with The Debrief that David Grusch is "beyond reproach.

David Grusch believes it is dangerous for this eighty-year arms race to continue in secrecy. He said it would "further inhibit the world populace to be prepared for un-expected, non-human intelligence contact scenario."

Just what does that mean when he says we may not be prepared for an un-expected non-human contact?

Does it mean the nations around the world will now acknowledge that there is an alien life form visiting planet earth, like the movie, The Day the Earth Stood Still?

Or does it mean non-human entities will attack us like "Independence Day?"

What is important are words and what they really mean. We have to look very closely at what is being said, how it's being said and what is being asked.

Grusch, who was very involved in the programs mentioned above, was asked if he had seen any of the photos of the alien crafts. He responded by saying, no he has not seen any photos of the crafts.

Of course how could that be true? We've all seen the photos that were plastered all over the media since 2017 which the Pentagon validated were true. However maybe not the crafts our government has in possession.

Another thought is Crusch was NGA's co-lead for UAP analysis and its representative to the task force. If he hadn't seen any pictures, then what was he analyzing? Was it just the money that was being allocated and to what programs?

However, He claims he has not seen any vehicles in person.

Given his involvement into these programs, it is almost inconceivable to believe he has not had any direct inter-action

Crusch did come out and say that what he witnessed was very disturbing.

If I was in that position, I would want to validate for myself these claims before I came forward.

It's important for the reader to know that government, especially top secret programs, work in what is called stove pipe departments. One program can be working in somewhat of the same arena as another program, collecting data, and not know what each other is doing or if they are even working in the same area. So if a department or program, like the AARO, (All Domain Anomaly Resolution Office), says they have no verifiable data of Grusch's claim, that may be true.

Although, NASA has come out and admitted they too have been involved.

However, Senator Marco Rubio, agrees there is more information out there. The Florida senator told <u>NewsNation</u> that others in addition to Grusch in the intelligence community have come forward with "firsthand" accounts of UFO hardware.

Rubio, an advocate for transparency on the alien issue, revealed that several more intelligence whistleblowers with "high clearances" have shared similar allegations as David Grusch with the Senate Intelligence Committee.

What we are finding is a deflection of who is being forth coming and who isn't.

One other concern I had during the congressional Intel hearings on UFO/UAPs, was the man sitting behind David Grusch. It appears to be James Clapper former director of National Intelligence. I personally believe James Clapper has lied to the American public. If you wish to review some of his lies and the reasons, it can be found here: [4 Different Lies James Clapper Told About Lying To Congress (thefederalist.com)](https://thefederalist.com)

Dishonesty and deception is an art that James Clapper seems to have mastered. It is a prerequisite for the CIA. It concerns me about the motive of why he would be there, if that is really him.

However, George Knapp of the Coast to Coast radio show was sitting next to him. George claims that it wasn't James Clapper but someone who looked like him.

I can believe that to be true and actually know for a fact, that there are people that look like each other. I have experienced this myself.

Whoever it is, could this all be a distraction from the political turmoil that is present at this writing?

These are the questions that must be asked.

Chapter 8

The Tom DeLonge connection.

Tom DeLonge, rock star and former founding member of the punk rock band "Blink 182 and founding member of Angels and Airwaves" had the ability to bring together a coalition of top people in science and government within his newly formed organization called "To the Star's Academy of Arts and Science."

His influence helped in the creation of the History Channel show called, *Unidentified* where former AATIP lead investigator Luis Elizondo helped document UFO/UAP sightings and encounters.

You may be asking, what does this all have to do with the Invisible Influence? It has everything to do with it because they are all connected.

Before the show was created, Tom Delonge came out and did some early interviews on the show called Coast to Coast and I shared some of my finding in my first book called "Out Of the Box Faith," which I will share here.

Out Of The Box Faith:

"Michael S. Heiser PhD, who was an ancient Hebrew language scholar, reveals in his book, "Hidden Realm" that Jehovah God had a council of divine beings (Ps 82) that he created with free will and those divine beings became rebellious; which in turn became the pagan gods' of the Old Testament and ancient mythology. He points out that the ancient people understood this and it was no shock to them. But this understanding has been clouded by our western world view and thus translated to fit that view.

On the other side of the demonic and angelic position, concerning UFOs, is Tom DeLonge, A.J. Hartley, Peter Levenda and many other very competent UFO researchers, who take a completely secular position on this topic. While there are other UFO researchers that have been in this field much longer, Tom DeLonge makes the claim that he has been researching this topic for many years and has had government assistance in attaining information about these beings.

Wiki Leaks revealed that Tom DeLonge and John Podesta (Hillary Clinton's advisor) actually had been working together on this topic of UFOs.

I listened to a 2 hour long interview with Tom DeLonge and hours of other interviews plus read his book's called: "Sekret Machines by Tom DeLonge and A.J. Hartley and book two, Gods, Man and War by Tom DeLonge and Peter Levenda."

Tom DeLonge points out that the first book, *Sekret Machines* is fiction. However he said that he obtained permission from the government to put it in this format to reveal things that are actually factual and real that our government is doing and where certain event actually happened.

When he says he received permission from the government, he pointed out that there is the government that we all know and openly see and then there is another side to the government that people never know about. Even within that other side of government there are stove pipe departments he claims to have been working with.

DeLonge reveals after years of research, an area of the government decided to work with him on the basis that they call the shots on what he can and cannot reveal.

He points out that the government doesn't call them aliens. They call them the "others." In this interview he said he was told that these "others" are responsible for what we know in historical mythology as, gods. These gods' that he is talking about claim that they are also responsible for all of the world's religions, even Christianity. These are the gods of mythology from the Mesopotamian, Greeks to the Egyptians and everything in between."

Tom DeLonge has jumped from books to his now new movie called *Monsters of California*. I believe the movie reveals a great deal of what took place within his family and the relationship he had with his mother in real life. And possibly who his father was and how he, as a musician, could accomplish a connection with our government on UFOs.

While the actors in the movie are fictional, the entities and events, according to Tom's early interviews, are very close to reality. The movie is entertaining with some harsh language and geared more toward reaching the youth.

The movie portrays the position that all things are connected: The paranormal, occult, ghosts and UFOs etc.

There's a connection of Tom DeLonge and the 2023 government whistle blower David Charles Grusch. They have something in common and as of this writing, no one seems to be connecting or at least not openly talking about it.

Tom DeLonge and David Crusch are revealing very much the same thing, yet years apart. What is that connection? That the United States government (or part of it) knows about these non-human entities and not only know about it, have alien crafts in their possession along with bodies.

Up until now, those I believe in the know, who have gone on the record, on shows like the History Channel of "Unidentified" make the claim they are trying to find out just what these UFO/UAPs are. When I believe in reality, they know what they are. Or maybe

I should say, they know what they believe they are, and know that our government has not only alien crafts, but back engineered technology and vehicles that we have built.

Also, back engineered technology may be responsible for the 2014 Malaysia flight 370 disappearance. More will be coming out about that.

Yet they give the impression they don't know what or who they are, when in fact it is highly probable, they do know but aren't allowed to reveal it in a published or public setting.

In 2016 Tom DeLonge pointed out in an interview that these beings that our government calls the "Others" have "god" like capabilities. What that means, I don't know.

Tom did point out that what they are able to do will be like magic to us.

He also pointed out that he believes when this all gets out or is revealed, it will "shake" the religious world to its core.

There are many other researchers that believe this to be true. He believes that when this information gets out, religions will be shaken to its core because they will realize, that these beings are the gods of their religion.

I wonder if this scripture addresses that kind shaking.

Heb 12:26-29

"Yet once more I will shake not only the earth but also the heavens." 27 This phrase, "Yet once more," indicates the removal of things that are shaken—that is, things that have been made—in order that the things that cannot be shaken may remain. 28 Therefore let us be grateful for receiving a kingdom that cannot be shaken, and thus let us offer to God acceptable worship, with reverence and awe, 29 for our God is a consuming fire." ESV

I can't help but wonder if the shaking of the religions that many of these researchers are referring too, mean people will lose their faith completely. That the revelation of these beings will shake loose their faith. And could this be what Jesus was referring too when he said: Luke 18:8

". . . when the Son of Man comes, will he find faith on earth?" ESV

Tom DeLonge shared that these entities that the government knows about uses mankind like chess pieces. They start conflict and wars. In order for them to do that, they have to influence the mindset of the world leaders.

Again this is in line with what George Knapp said when he was informed by someone high up in government that these beings manipulate mankind and cause wars.

The logical conclusion is, if that happens, it's done by the influence of the mind in the world leaders.

Tom DeLonge no longer mentions what he knows or what he has shared in the past interviews.

Even on the History Channel show *Unidentified*, he gave the appearance as though he didn't know what the UFO/UAPs were.

I suspect that his government handlers told him to stop or slow down in revealing what he knows.

He also pointed out that our government is spending huge amounts of money for a possible conflict in the future against some of these entities.

I don't know if that is a seed to lay out there for a possible false flag in order to garner more money for the vast industrial military complex or not, but it would not surprise me if that was the motivation.

Or it could be something that could try and unite the world behind a one world government. Time will tell.

Where are they getting this huge amount of money? Could it be the billions or trillions that government seem to lose every few years?

This may or may not be the false flag that I've been hearing about concerning UFOs. It may be something to deflect ones attention away from the political turmoil; a diversion to look over here and not there?

Wars and rumors of wars also deflect from the political hardship someone may be facing.

Regardless, there seems to be a building of momentum in the revealing of UFO's and to convince people that they are real and have been with us for many years.

Just the opposite of what our government has been telling us and hiding for some 80 plus years. Yet there are still those in government that don't want any of this to get out.

Whether it is a false flag or not, the issue of UFO's are real. Top ranking officials are going on record to say just that. This from the Debrief article by Leslie Kean and Ralph Blumenthal, June 5th 2023:

"Jonathan Grey is a generational officer of the United States Intelligence Community with a Top-Secret Clearance who currently works for the National Air and Space Intelligence Center (NASIC), where the analysis of UAP has been his focus. Previously he had experience serving Private Aerospace and Department of Defense Special Directive Task Forces."

"The non-human intelligence phenomenon is real. We are not alone," Grey said. "Retrievals of this kind are not limited to the United States. This is a global phenomenon, and yet a global solution continues to elude us."

Jonathan Grey says secrets have been necessary. "Though a tough nut to crack, potential technological advancements may be gleaned from non-human intelligence/UAP retrievals by any sufficiently advanced nation and then used to wage asymmetrical warfare, so, therefore, some secrecy must remain," he says. "However, it is no longer necessary to continue to deny that these advanced technologies derived from non-human intelligence exist at all or to deny that these technologies have landed, crashed, or fallen into the hands of human beings."

Some of the people that are connected to our government may in fact know what Tom DeLonge and David Grusch know and give the appearance that they are looking into this issue of UFO/UAPs but don't really know what or who they are.

Could this method of, 'I don't know what they are' be a form of controlled disclosure?

My suspicion is, those that are close to Tom DeLonge know the same as he knows, yet pretending they don't know much about what the UFO/UAPs are but are trying to find out.

Chapter 9

Global Manipulation by Non-Human Influence

If you have read down this far you know that the premise of my position is that the elites of our world (a small number of non-elected people) are in fact directing many of the nation's leaders, including the U.S.A. through the United Nations, WHO (World Health Organization) and the WEF (World Economic Forum). The Trinity of government control.

As Tom DeLonge stated in his early interviews that these non-human entities use humans as chest pieces and have been manipulating mankind.

George Knapp who broke the news of the Area 51 back in the 1980s and one of the hosts of the nation-wide radio show Coast to Coast made the same claim, that mankind is being manipulated.

These non-human entities that influence mankind, heads of state and the elites of our world, are far more intelligent and shrewder than any individual upon this earth.

Their goal is not to eliminate man-kind completely, but to control and change what it means to be human and to reduce the population down to a sustainable and controllable number, to bring the world under a single controlling power through the United Nations spear headed by the WEF - global reset. (Agenda 2030 - 2050)

When I say change what it means to be human, that is exactly what they are saying. They are simply saying, as humans you are now hackable, just like a computer/machine.

Even though many have high praises for Elon Musk, he has what is called the neural-lace project that merges man and machine through the brain.

What it does is merges biological intelligence with machine intelligence. The effort on one hand is to make you better, in what way we don't know yet, but also, to correct medical issues people may have.

We have to ask, what will it do? Will it make it possible for them to manipulate you in a direction you may not ordinarily go?

Then we have Yuval Harari. Harari is a history professor at the Hebrew University in Jerusalem. He's wrote 3 books that have sold over 35 million in 65 languages.

In the article called *The Sociable* March 16th 2022 it says, "Harari warned that humans were no longer mysterious soul, but rather hackable animals that could be monitored and controlled by public and private entities ...."

Harari also said, "Just imagine North Korea in 20 years where everybody has to wear a biometric bracelet, which constantly monitors your blood pressure, you heart rate, your brain activity 24 hours a day. You listen to a speech on the radio by the "Great Leader," and they know what you actually feel - you can clap your hands and smile, but if you're angry, they know you'll be in the gulag tomorrow morning – Yuval Harari, WEF, 2020."

Harari said, companies and world leaders, believe those who control the most data will control the world.

This technology to hack humans is now in development by (DARPA) and the program is called NEAT (Neural Evidence Aggregation Tool). It is a cognitive science tool and the goal is to determine what you believe to be true or false, and the government or the controlling power in charge, will know it, but also if you are at risk of suicide.

<u>Yuval Noah Harari: 'Homo sapiens as we know them will disappear in a century or so' | Yuval Noah Harari | The Guardian</u>

Harari also said '... we are in danger of becoming an elite-dominated global society.'

While there may not seem to be a connection, there is also the question of the Covid19 vaccine changing your DNA. Some argue it doesn't. Other say it has been proven that it does. Some say it is actually gene alteration.

We do know those that are in support of the vaccines have lied about its effectiveness from the beginning. Are we to believe them now when they say it doesn't change your DNA?

Some are saying that the mRNA (m) standing for messenger, is NOT messenger at all but rather (m) stands for modified. And if modified, many believe this is why the shot doesn't remain in the arm location but moves throughout the body.

There is still a lot to be learned by what has been a deception by our government and medical industry.

It is the focus of what is taking place to take control of our world and bring it under a central power like the U.N.

The agenda 2030 by the UN in their listed goals, there is NO mention or room for people of faith. Faith, religion or belief in a creator is nowhere mentioned in their declarations that I could find.

While the agenda of a basic one world controlling power has been in the planning for many years there has been an implementation starting in 2016 toward that goal.

"21. The new Goals and targets will come into effect on 1 January 2016 and will guide the decisions we take over the next fifteen years. All of us will work to implement the Agenda within our own countries and at the regional and global levels, taking into account different national realities, capacities and levels of development and respecting national policies and priorities. We will respect national policy space for sustained, inclusive and sustainable economic growth, in particular for developing states, while remaining consistent with relevant international rules and commitments. We acknowledge also the importance of the regional and sub-regional dimensions, regional economic integration and interconnectivity in sustainable development. Regional and sub-regional frameworks can facilitate the effective translation of sustainable development policies into concrete action at national level."

Sustainable development policies must be achieved. What does that mean? The answer is, it means a reduction in consumption of food and population. To control from a central world government.

Now comes the realization of what has been taking place that seem irrational to the average person.

The present Democratic administration and the deep state Republicans in America believes in the global warming or now called Climate Change, of impending doom, if something isn't done soon; ignoring the past fifty years of false climate catastrophe warnings.

<u>50 Years of Failed Doomsday, Eco-pocalyptic Predictions; the So-called 'experts' Are 0-50 | American Enterprise Institute - AEI</u>

The invisible influence that help guide those in charge to bring about conditions that will appear natural in nature but are manufactured is all in the preparation of establishing control.

The Biden administration has warned of the coming food shortages.

During and shortly after president Biden's warning of food shortages we had for the first time in our nation's history a massive number of food processing plants burn and shut down all within one years' time. How is that possible?

Here is a list:

LIST OF DESTROYED U.S. FOOD PROCESSING FACILITIES:

The Gateway Pundit provided the following list of destroyed American food manufacturing sites:

1/11/21 A fire destroyed a 75,000-square-foot processing plant in Fayetteville

4/30/21 A fire started inside the Smithfield Foods pork processing plant in Monmouth, IL

7/25/21 Three-alarm fire at Kellogg plant in Memphis, 170 emergency personnel responded to the call

7/30/21 Firefighters battled a large fire at Tyson's River Valley Ingredients plant in Hanceville, Alabama

8/23/21 Fire crews were called to the Patak Meat Production company on Ewing Road in Austell

9/13/21 A fire at the JBS beef plant in Grand Island, Neb., forced a halt to slaughter and fabrication lines

10/13/21 A five-alarm fire demolished the Darigold butter production plant in Caldwell, ID

11/15/21 A woman is in custody following a fire at the Garrard County Food Pantry

11/29/21 A fire began around 5:30 p.m. at the Maid-Rite Steak Company meat processing plant

12/13/21 West Side food processing plant in San Antonio left with smoke damage after a fire

1/7/22 Damage to a poultry processing plant on Hamilton's Mountain following an overnight fire

1/13/22 Firefighters worked for 12 hours to put a fire out at the Cargill-Nutrena plant in Lecompte, LA

1/31/22 A fertilizer plant with 600 tons of ammonium nitrate inside caught on fire on Cherry Street in Winston-Salem

2/3/22 A massive fire swept through Wisconsin River Meats in Mauston

2/3/22 At least 130 cows were killed in a fire at Percy Farm in Stowe

2/15/22 Bonanza Meat Company goes up in flames in El Paso, Texas

2/15/22 Nearly a week after the fire destroyed most of the Shearer's Foods plant in Hermiston

2/16/22 A fire had broken at the largest US soybean processing and biodiesel plant in Claypool, Indiana

2/18/22 An early morning fire tore through the milking parlor at Bess View Farm

2/19/22 Three people were injured, and one was hospitalized, after an ammonia leak at Lincoln Premium Poultry in Fremont

2/22/22 The Shearer's Foods plant in Hermiston caught fire after a propane boiler exploded

2/28/22 A smoldering pile of sulfur quickly became a raging chemical fire at Nutrien Ag Solutions

2/28/22 A man was hurt after a fire broke out at the Shadow Brook Farm and Dutch Girl Creamery

3/4/22 294,800 chickens destroyed at a farm in Stoddard, Missouri

3/4/22 644,000 chickens destroyed at egg farm in Cecil, Maryland

3/8/22 243,900 chickens destroyed at egg farm in New Castle, Delaware

3/10/22 663,400 chickens destroyed at egg farm in Cecil, MD

3/10/22 915,900 chickens destroyed at egg farm in Taylor, IA

3/14/22 The blaze at 244 Meadow Drive was discovered shortly after 5 p.m. by farm owner Wayne Hoover

3/14/22 2,750,700 chickens destroyed at egg farm in Jefferson, Wisconsin

3/16/22 A fire at a Walmart warehouse distribution center in Plainfield, Indiana has cast a large plume of smoke visible throughout Indianapolis.

3/16/22 Nestle Food Plant extensively damaged in fire and new production destroyed Jonesboro, Arkansas

3/17/22 5,347,500 chickens destroyed at egg farm in Buena Vista, Iowa

3/17/22 147,600 chickens destroyed at farm in Kent, Delaware

3/18/22 315,400 chickens destroyed at egg farm in Cecil, Maryland

3/22/22 172,000 Turkeys destroyed on farms in South Dakota

3/22/22 570,000 chickens destroyed at farm in Butler, Nebraska

3/24/22 Fire fighters from numerous towns are battling a major fire at the McCrum potato processing facility in Belfast, Maine.

3/24/22 418,500 chickens destroyed at farm in Butler, Nebraska

3/25/22 250,300 chickens destroyed at egg farm in Franklin, Iowa

3/26/22 311,000 Turkeys destroyed in Minnesota

3/27/22 126,300 Turkeys destroyed in South Dakota

3/28/22 1,460,000 chickens destroyed at egg farm in Guthrie, Iowa

3/29/22 A massive fire burned 40,000 pounds of food meant to feed people in a food desert near Maricopa

3/31/22 A structure fire caused significant damage to a large portion of key fresh onion packing facilities in south Texas

3/31/22 76,400 Turkeys destroyed in Osceola, Iowa

3/31/22 5,011,700 chickens destroyed at egg farm in Osceola, Iowa

4/6/22 281,600 chickens destroyed at farm in Wayne, North Carolina

4/9/22 76,400 Turkeys destroyed in Minnesota

4/9/22 208,900 Turkeys destroyed in Minnesota

4/12/22 89,700 chickens destroyed at farm in Wayne, North Carolina

4/12/22 1,746,900 chickens destroyed at egg farm in Dixon, Nebraska

4/12/22 259,000 chickens destroyed at farm in Minnesota

4/13/22 Fire destroys East Conway Beef & Pork Meat Market in Conway, New Hampshire

4/13/22 Plane crashes into Gem State Processing, Idaho potato and food processing plant

4/13/22 77,000 Turkeys destroyed in Minnesota

4/14/22 Taylor Farms Food Processing plant burns down Salinas, California.

4/14/22 99,600 Turkeys destroyed in Minnesota

4/15/22 1,380,500 chickens destroyed at egg farm in Lancaster, Minnesota

4/19/22 Azure Standard nation's premier independent distributor of organic and healthy food, was destroyed by fire in Dufur, Oregon

4/19/22 339,000 Turkeys destroyed in Minnesota

4/19/22 58,000 chickens destroyed at farm in Montrose, Color

4/20/22 2,000,000 chickens destroyed at egg farm in Minnesota

4/21/22 A small plane crashed in the lot of a General Mills plant in Covington, Georgia

4/22/22 197,000 Turkeys destroyed in Minnesota
4/23/22 200,000 Turkeys destroyed in Minnesota
4/25/22 1,501,200 chickens destroyed at egg farm Cache, Utah
4/26/22 307,400 chickens destroyed at farm Lancaster Pennsylvania
4/27/22 2,118,000 chickens destroyed at farm Knox, Nebraska
4/28/22 Egg-laying facility in Iowa kills 5.3 million chickens, fires 200-plus workers
4/28/22 Allen Harim Foods processing plant killed nearly 2M chickens in Delaware
4/2822 110,700 Turkeys destroyed Barron Wisconsin
4/29/22 5 million honeybees are dead after a flight carrying the pollinator insects from California to Alaska got diverted to Georgia (New)
4/29/22 1,366,200 chickens destroyed at farm Weld Colorado
4/30/22 13,800 chickens destroyed at farm Sequoia Oklahoma
5/3/22 58,000 Turkeys destroyed Barron Wisconsin
5/3/22 118,900 Turkeys destroyed Beadle S Dakota
5/3/22 114,000 ducks destroyed at Duck farm Berks Pennsylvania
5/3/22 118,900 Turkeys destroyed Lyon Minnesota
5/7/22 20,100 Turkeys destroyed Barron Wisconsin
5/10/22 72,300 chickens destroyed at a farm Lancaster Pennsylvania
5/10/22 61,000 ducks destroyed at Duck farm Berks Pennsylvania
5/10/22 35,100 Turkeys destroyed Muskegon, Michigan
5/13/22 10,500 Turkeys destroyed Barron Wisconsin

5/14/22 83,400 ducks destroyed at Duck farm Berks Pennsylvania

5/17/22 79,00 chickens destroyed at Duck farm Berks Pennsylvania

5/18/22 7,200 ducks destroyed at Duck farm Berks Pennsylvania

5/19/22 Train carrying limestone derailed Jensen Beach FL

5/21/22 57,000 Turkeys destroyed on farm in Dakota Minnesota

5/23/22 4,000 ducks destroyed at Duck farm Berks Pennsylvania

5/29/22 A Saturday night fire destroyed a poultry building at Forsman Farms in Howard Lake, Minnesota

5/31/22 3,000,000 chickens destroyed by fire at Forsman facility in Stockholm Township, Minnesota

6/2/22 30,000 ducks destroyed at Duck farm Berks Pennsylvania

6/7/22 A fire occurred Tuesday evening at the JBS meat packing plant in Green Bay, Wisconsin

6/8/22 Firefighters from Tangipahoa Fire District 1 respond to a fire at the Purina Feed Mill in Arcola, Louisiana

6/9/22 Irrigation water was canceled in California (the #1 producer of food in the US) and storage water flushed directly out to the delta.

6/12/22 Largest pork company in the US shuts down California plant due to high costs

6/13/22 Fire broke out at a food processing plant west of Waupaca County in Wisconsin

6/14/22 Over 10,000 head of cattle have reportedly died in the recent Kansas heat wave

6/23/22 George's Inc.: Poultry and Prepared Foods announced it will close one of its food processing plants in Campbell County, Tennessee

8/10/22 A fire completely destroyed a building at Pendleton Flour Mills in Eastern Oregon

8/28/22 A poultry processing plant in Montebello, California caught on fire

8/30/22 An emergency was declared in four states after an oil refinery fire in Indiana disrupted the supply of gasoline, diesel, and jet fuel

What is taking place are leaders following the direction of a small number of elites (influenced by non-human entities) found within the United Nations and the now (WEF) Great Reset, and are finding ways to fulfill their predictions of coming calamities. They predict it, then make it happen.

They are working to change the way we eat and how they supply us with food.

"28. We commit to making fundamental changes in the way that our societies produce and consume goods and services.

These 14 US Cities Have A 'Target' Of Banning Meat By 2030 (thefederalist.com)

C40 Cities is the NEW WORLD ORDER and CLIMATE CHANGE push of the Agenda 2030.

Bill Gates has invested in lab grown meat and why he is now the largest private farm land owner in America.

Outside of corporations the largest farm land owner is the "Church of the Jesus Christ - Latter Day Saints, Mormon," then Bill Gates.

Just as they are predicting the next pandemic, (as Anthony Fauci did in 2017 right before Trump took office) they already have their planning in the works to make the food pandemic and other future pandemics, happen. This is why Bill Gates and others are coming out and talking about the next pandemic to come. They seem to always telegraph their action.

In Belgium Bill Gate is predicting what he calls a catastrophic contagion in or around 2025. They even have a name for the contagion called, SEERS which stands for, Sever Epidemic Entrovirus Respiratory Syndrome 2025.

China calls their newly developed virus, diseaseX and will have a very high kill rate.

[Amid elites' talk of 'Disease X,' Chinese lab debuts mutant coronavirus with 100% kill rate in humanized mice | Blaze Media (theblaze.com)](#)

According to this next pandemic prediction it will kill over 20 million, infect possibly hundreds of million children leaving many of them brain damaged.

This is what DiseaseX is reported to do is attack the brain and the lungs among other parts of our organs.

According to them they will have a "vaccine" to combat this pandemic. <u>Make NO mistake, this is what they are planning to make happen in one form or another.</u>

The fear will increase and they will once again gain greater control and strip away freedoms because the people will allow it.

<u>It's starting, Bill Gates announces the next pandemic date and outbreak location | Redacted News - YouTube</u>

People will once again trust in their government not just because of fear, but because they will use words that will comfort them into compliance.

On top of all this the United Nations agenda 2030 claims they will eliminate world poverty. Sounds wonderful, doesn't it? Using words that sound good to people, but will ultimately have a nefarious outcome.

Jesus said, the poor you will always have. So how do they plan to do that without lowering the population?

Robert Kennedy Jr said that it is an insane proposal to think we are capable of eliminating the poor or poverty in the world.

There's a difference between helping the poor and eliminating the poor. But that is exactly what the United Nations is proposing.

Many will have open arms to what the United Nations and the WEF (World Economic Forum) are doing, because it all sounds good and helpful.

Bate & Switch

When deception is effective it means the one deceiving you was able to convince you of something that isn't what you think it is.

When speaking of those promoting the Agenda 2030 and the Great Reset, we're saying they use language that will make you feel good about their intentions.

They use words that will sway and convince you that their goal is for your betterment. What they are not telling you, their goal is to reduce the population, eliminate private property and to place you in what they call a sustainable city, now being called 15 minute cities. Great changes will have to happen for it to be completed and they are working toward that right now.

The current U.S. president Joe Biden is wanting people to reduce or eliminate natural gas appliances and to go all electric plus pushing to eliminate or limit gas vehicles. This at a time where many states are struggling to maintain their electrical grid.

It's about controlling almost every aspect of your life. Even the speed you drive your car.

Cars to be programmed to limit speed if California bill becomes law | Frontline News

Once you move to all electric they will have greater control over your use once the social credit score is implemented.

Leaders like Governor Gavin Newsom of California and Michelle Lujan Grisham, governor of New Mexico, is following the WEF/United Nation agenda 2030 goals by eliminating gas cars. This under the idea of sustainable energy resource. Which is actually the opposite of what it will accomplish.

"Today, the California Air Resources Board voted to only allow the sale of new passenger cars, trucks, and SUVs in California if they have zero tailpipe emissions, starting in **2035**. Passage of the Advanced Clean Cars II (ACCII) proposal means no new gas-engine vehicles and no new diesels will be sold in the state a dozen years from now."

Going all electric is a disastrous plan and unachievable. However the more they can transfer you over to the electric grid, the sooner they can control your energy needs and you.

If another governor that takes Newsom's place and follows in line with this agenda it may be moved up sooner than 2035. But you'll not need a car anyways because you'll be living in what they call sustainable 15 minute cities.

15 Minute cities is where you will have no need for cars, and you'll be within 15 minutes of services or work. You will either walk to your destination or they will have public transportation. Everything will be provide for you by the government, even your housing; as long as your social credit score is on the positive side. You will rent everything from the government.

In Klaus Schwab's "Covid19 The Great Rest" some critics attribute the saying "you'll own nothing and be happy" to Klaus Schwab. But the phrase **originated** by Danish **Politician Ida Auken in a 2016 essay for the World Economic Forum (WEF)** which Klaus Schwab is the head of.

Yet it is part of the stated goal. You will own nothing and you'll be happy is what they are working to accomplish. You will see in a later Chapter how this is a new spin on a Marxist principle.

Chapter 10

Global Population Reduction

As we mentioned in the previous chapter concerning staged pandemics. Who for the purpose of controlling the world population, must do it in a way that you don't suspect what their goals are.

They depend upon your ignorance. Thomas Jefferson said:

"If a nation expects to be ignorant and free, in a state of civilization, it expects what never was and never will be."

War has always been a good way of reducing the population and no one suspects.

The advancement in biotech has added a new and unsuspecting dimension of reducing the population, while at the same time making people believe they are being helped. All through the medical field.

Who always telegraph their intentions in a way that will sound reasonable and needed.

In order for you to accept the idea of population reduction they must convince you that the population of the earth is unsustainable and somehow man must find a way to reduce the population in order for mankind to survive.

Behind many of the elites is the little known name of Pepe Orisi. As I stated earlier many believe Pepe Orisi to be what they call the gray pope and wheels a great deal of power and influence throughout the world and has a long blood line within the Holy Roman Papal.

Pepe Orisi is also known to be a major de-populationist and is believed to be working with the black pope which is also called the Jesuits general.

There is a spider web of connections

. in the Vatican and among the elites and all appear to be working in the same direction.

An article by Britta DeVore 8/18/23 titled: "Scientist Say A Terrifying Population Correction Is Coming."

<u>Scientists Say A Terrifying Population Correction Is Coming Soon (msn.com)</u>

Here is first two paragraphs:

"As if we didn't have enough to worry about between the spooky and downright unsettling raise of artificial intelligence and global warming, scientists are now warning that the earth's population is getting out of control.

This shouldn't necessarily come as a surprise as it's not exactly new news, but population ecologist William Rees of the University of British Columbia in Canada (as per science alert) is now coming forward to say there may be a dire need for a population correction. As terrifying as that sounds, the move could point to extreme consequences over the next few decades."

More evidence that they are expecting something to bring down or slow down the world population.

Dr. James Hill reported on what is called the Deagel.com which is from the Deagel Corporation and is often used by our military and forecast as early as 2014 future events, predicts up to 80% of the population culled by 2025 in countries where Europeans live.

On their chart it also shows in America where we stand at 332 million as of 2023 will possibly drop down to 99 million by 2025 or a few years later. That is a 70.2 percent drop.

Deagel.com predicts up to 80% of population culled by 2025 in countries where Europeans live (substack.com)

Why are they predicting this? Or is it a prediction by plan?

For that prediction to come to fruition the only thing I could think of in eliminating some 200 million plus in such a very short time would be a nuclear strike upon America or a deadly virus called DiseaseX? They may indeed have other ways that is out of our ability to comprehend.

So we have to ask, just what mechanism is going to drop the world population in such a dramatic rate? Wars? Bio-Pandemics? Could it be a combination of both?

There are news articles here and there that point to the same sentiment about being over populated.

Many commentators are fearful of even going down that rabbit hole for fear of sounding like an extremist. Yet in the back of their minds, they know something is brewing in that direction.

The scary part isn't them talking about depopulation. The scary part, voiced by many medical professionals is, they've already started the process through various types of pandemics, wars and many believe vaccines are included in that scenario.

Data out of New Zealand from a whistle blower, implies worldwide over 13 - 17 million have died from the Covid19 vaccine alone.

The sad part is the New Zealand government has tried to silence this whistle blower by throwing him in jail.

Let me give a disclaimer here. If you've received the Covid19 vaccine and boosters, you will receive no condemnation or rebuke from me nor should you feel guilty. You did what you thought was right. All of us, whether we were vaccinated or not, were deceived by our government and health departments officials under the direction of the NIH and CDC.

We all wanted to believe that what our government was telling us was the truth. However, our government lied to us and continues to lie to us.

I have family and friends who were misled and took these shots they call vaccines; some who were injured and a very close friend of mine who died.

Many medical professionals and others believe it wasn't just the Covid19 virus that is the population controller, it was and still is, the Covid19 vaccine using the mRNA and boosters that could not pass the standard testing protocols.

Many opposition voices in the medical field believe the Covid19 vaccines and boosters to be one of the population reduction tools that will be felt years into the future.

Who are even working to put the mRNA into our food products and livestock and to possibly aerosolize the mRNA to vaccinate everyone without their permission by spraying it in the air. Why?

To force it upon people without their permission means they have an ulterior, and I believe, nefarious motive.

On top of all this, Bill Gates said, "The world today has 6.8 billion people. That's headed up to about 9 billion. Now, if we do a really great job on **new vaccines**, health care, reproductive health services (Abortions, my word), we could lower that by, perhaps, 10 or 15%."

Many of us who heard what he said, find it hard to believe, that they can actually lower the population through vaccines.

He explains that when people are healthier they choose to have less children, thus a lower population. You can hear him explain that here. Does saving more lives lead to overpopulation? - YouTube

There might be evidence for his claim; although I couldn't find any. The only problem is, the first observable (antidotal) evidence from Covid19 vaccines are doing just the opposite and doing what we all think when we hear about lowering the population through "vaccines."

There is now documentation that the vaccines are in fact having the opposite reaction and not making you healthier.

Not only are they killing people from the vaccines at an unprecedented rate, they are injuring millions of people which means the health of individuals are being lowered and possible early deaths. So it is having the opposite effect of what he claims.

Remember what I said about them (the elite, government and mainstream news and media platforms) using words that make you believe in one direction, when in fact, they mean just the opposite.

Bill Gates may be using the excuse that when people are healthier they have less children and that lowers the population. But the Covid-vaccines/boosters are in fact validating our suspicions that it is the vaccines themselves depopulating.

Life insurance companies said since the vaccine came out, they called it apocalyptic in life-insurance claims that they never expected or predicted.

And again, why are they trying to force us to take the vaccines when the evidence is so clear? Has our freedom of choice been removed?

Trying to Hide

Pfizer Company had asked a judge to keep their documents on the vaccine and procedures hidden for 75 years.

Now if you're a person who has a rational mind knows that if they're wanting to hide what is in the vaccine and what it was doing to people in some of their early phase testing for 75 years, you know it's not something that will be good or beneficial for mankind.

However the judge in their case said no you cannot keep those files hidden for 75 years. So they did release some of the documents.

Naomi Wolf, who is a lifelong Democratic journalist and feminist asked medical professionals to help decipher the some 55 thousand pages of Pfizer documents.

From that call, she got over 2,500 experts then growing to 3,200 from around the world offering to help her in deciphering the medical jargon within those 55 thousand pages and more.

They were professionals from almost every field within the range of understanding these documents. Then she got an offer from a woman by the name of Amy Kelly who offered to be Naomi Wolf's project manager and to coordinate the different areas of expertise.

She produced reports based off these primary source documents so they could, through these reports from highly skilled experts in their field, share with the world just what was in these documents and the possible dangers related to them.

From that time they produced 85 reports as of this writing. According to Naomi Wolf, <u>she believes the greatest crime against humanity are found in these documents.</u> Which again, supports our suspicions that Bill Gates believes that the vaccines will reduce the population and not through being healthier.

Pfizer knew one month after the roll out of the vaccines, 2020 that the vaccines did not stop Covid19 infection and continued to lie, with the help of our government, social and mainstream media, to the public.

One of the points that stand out in what they found was, the third most common side effect of getting the vaccine was, you came down with Covid19. Some who got the boosters came down with Covid several times.

Pfizer knew in May of 2021 that the vaccine cause heart damage in 35 minors within a week of getting the vaccine.

<u>What's in the Pfizer Documents? | Naomi Wolf - Bing video</u>

Dr. Robert Malone who is one of the original inventors of the mRNA research is calling on the government to stop all Covid19 vaccines and boosters for the variants. Dr. Malone was injured himself from the Covid19 vaccine.

Dr. Robert Malone said "Over the last 3 years you have been subjected to the most massive harmonized globally coordinated propaganda campaign in the history of the western world, full stop. With this campaign the governments of many western nation state have turned, this is key, military grade psychological operations strategies tactics and technologies and capabilities developed for modern military combat against their own citizens. These are inconvenient facts … that many of us believed existed no longer exist, if it ever did. Welcome to fifth-generation warfare. The battle field is your MIND."

Again, Dr. Robert Malone along with Dr. Peter McCullough and many other highly respected professionals within the medical community have been de-plat-formed by social media and silenced because they held an opposing position from our government.

So we have to ask. What or who influences people, heads of states and institutions to commit such atrocities by secretly committing acts that would reduce the population?

This type of action isn't knew. In the 1970s when our government went to the Native American reservations and using "free health care" sterilizing the women (coercing and sometimes unknowingly to them) so they couldn't reproduce.

Native Americans, government authorities, and reproductive politics : News Center (rochester.edu)

You had The Tuskegee Experiment of African-American's in the 1930s.

Then you had **The Aversion Project**

They didn't like gay people in apartheid-era South Africa. Especially in the armed forces. How they got rid of them is shocking. Using army psychiatrists and military chaplains, who were, presumably privy to private, "confidential" confessions, the apartheid regime flushed out homosexuals in the armed forces. But it did not evict them from the military. The homosexual "undesirables" were sent to a military hospital near Pretoria, to a place called Ward 22 (which in itself sounds terrifying).

There, between 1971 and 1989, many victims were submitted to chemical castrations and electric shock treatment, meant to cure them of their homosexual "condition." As many as 900 homosexuals, mostly 16-24 years old who had been drafted and had not voluntarily joined the military, were subjected to forced "sexual reassignment" surgeries. Men were surgically made to appear as a women against their will, then cast out into the world, the gender reassignment often incomplete, and without the means to pay for expensive hormones to maintain their new sexual identities.

10 of the Most Evil Medical Experiments Conducted in History - Alternet.org

The point is, government who we believe to be there to protect and serve, is often the purveyor of evil in our world.

As I mentioned earlier. Non-human entities plant thoughts and ideas and then the snowball effect takes place. Using the darker side of human nature where it becomes a planned agenda.

Chapter 11

The Chest Piece scenario

As Tom DeLonge pointed out in one of his earlier interviews, that these entities have not only been here since the origins of man upon this earth. They have been using mankind as chest pieces and manipulating their thinking processes; creating conflicts, wars and policies of nations that continue to bring its citizens under greater control.

As I have mentioned in the previous Chapter about the many gods of the past and how they have influenced their nations and culture.

List of Gods and Goddesses From Antiquity (learnreligions.com)

It is important to recognize that these entities (some may call demons others call them aliens) influence individuals who in turn bring about great change.

One person who has had his influence upon the past and now our current world today, and I believe for the future, was Carl Marx.

Marxism can be dressed up in many different ways, but it's still Marxism in principle, and if society or a nation is ignorant to his political and philosophical positions, they will fall prey to its historical consequences.

Carl Marx, known for Marxism, is also the author of the Communist manifesto.

His political philosophies are antithetical to Christian and honest-capitalist principles and history is replete with the failures of those positions he held.

What people may not know or realize, Carl Marx had 6 points that actually destroys the western world culture and our American way of life. Those principles are being implemented through the WEF (World Economic Forum) and in many ways, through our American system today. To advance Marxist objectives, it must be done incrementally and done in a way that appeals to the masses to go along with the reshaped Marxist principles, or by coercion.

Here are some of his primary positions:

1. *Abolition of Private Property.*

Carl Marx was famous for his Communist Manifesto. Marx's ideas are very much like what the WEF (World

Economic Forum) and the Covid19, Great Reset that Klaus Schwab talks about, to "eliminate private property." Thus, the statement of "You will own nothing, and be happy." This will apply to all, even the upper middle class.

Carl Marx said, "To sum up Communism, is the abolition of private property."

2. *Family.*
Carl Marx was astonishingly honest about his positions. When the topic of family comes up, Marx was completely frank about his position. He said destroying the family was a thorny topic, even for revolutionaries. "Abolition of the family! He said opponents of this idea fail to understand a key fact about the family. "On what foundation is the present family, the bourgeois (middle class) family, based? His battle was class warfare.

He went on to say it was on capital, on private gain. In its completely developed form, this family exists only among the bourgeoisie, (meaning the middle class). Best of all, abolishing the family would be relatively easy once bourgeois (middle class) property was abolished. "The bourgeois (middle class) family will vanish as a matter of course when its complement vanishes, and both will vanish with the vanishing of capital."

Marx ideas of destroying the middle class was central to his political position. Take private property away and eliminate the middle class through eliminating the capitalist system which also, in his mind, eliminates middle class families. Government will own everything. That is where he felt unity and cohesiveness resides, in government who owns all and takes care of all its citizens. Very much like our Democrat and Deep State Republican Party today through the expansion of government. It's done all at once. It's done incrementally.

3. Individuality

Carl Marx held the position that individuality was antithetical to egalitarianism (the idea that all are equal). Therefore, the idea of "individual" must "be eliminated, and made impossible."

This very idea is what the WEF (World Economic Forum) is trying to promote through the idea of "it takes a village to raise a child" or communitarianism. Instead of individualism and personal responsibility; it promotes collectivism where individualism is not a focus but rather a community that owns nothing and ruled by the government.

Marx believed that individuality was a social construct of a capitalist society and was deeply intertwined with capital itself.

Carl Marx believed the middle class society capital makes a person independent and has individuality, while the living or what he called the working person, is dependent and has no individuality.

For Marx the abolition of the (middle class), would help to eliminate individuality and ultimately the freedom it gave the middle class! He believed that it was good to eliminate those freedoms by eliminating capitalism.

The elimination of the (middle class) individuality, private property, independence, and freedoms without a doubt is the aim of the WEF.

4. *Eternal Truths*

It appears that Marx did not believe any truth existed beyond what he considered, class struggle.

Carl Marx said: "The ruling ideas of each age have ever been the ideas of its ruling class." He went on to say: "When the ancient world was in its last throes, the ancient religions were overcome by Christianity. When Christian ideas succumbed in the 18th century to rationalist ideas, feudal (combination of legal, economic, cultural and political customs) society fought its death battle with the then revolutionary bourgeoisie (middle class)."

Marx believed that Communism does not seek to modify truth, but to overthrow it. Marx knew this and he knew how far-reaching it sounded. But he argued these people were missing the larger picture.

"'Undoubtedly,' it will be said, 'religious, moral, philosophical, and juridical ideas have been modified in the course of historical development. But religion, morality, philosophy, political science, and law, constantly survived this change.

There is no doubt that eternal truths, such as Freedom, Justice, etc., are common to all states of society. However, Communism abolishes eternal truths, <u>it abolishes all religion</u>, and all morality, instead of constituting them on a new basis; it therefore acts in contradiction to all past historical experience."

What does this all really mean? Marx continues: "The history of all past society has consisted in the development of class antagonisms, antagonisms that assumed different forms at different epochs."

Marx believed that the upper class, in this case, middle class, held down those below and to correct what he believed was injustice, the middle class and the freedoms that came along with it, had to be eliminated in order to produce the greater good, in his opinion.

A side note here. Today many of our politicians, while not openly proclaiming they are Communists/Marxists, adopt the principles of eliminating enteral truths of morality. Like, lying to accomplish their political goals or to besmirch an opponent or to simply talk about defending the constitution while actually tearing it down. It's all about deception and manipulation because truth is over thrown.

5. *Nations*

Carl Marx said Communists are reproached for seeking to abolish countries. Communism is the idea of all being under one central control. (Thus, the idea of One World Government) Marx felt people fail to understand the nature of the proletariat (working man).

Marx says: "The working men have no country. We cannot take from them what they have not got. Since the proletariat (working man) must first of all acquire political supremacy, must rise to be the leading class of the nation, must constitute itself the nation, it is so far, itself national, though not in the bourgeois (middle class) sense of the word."

Meaning, if the working man gains power and position, like the middle class, it's not the same, because he started out as a working man (Proletariat). It is a perverse form of logic.

Due to capitalism where people were escaping poverty, he could see hostilities between people of different backgrounds receding. As the proletariat (working man) grew in power, he felt there might not be any need for nations.

Marx looked at the working man gaining power as a dichotomy. It's not the same for a working man to gain power as those who already belong to the middle class. (It's mental gymnastics to justify his irrational position).

Marx could see that national differences and antagonism between peoples were vanishing, owing it to the development of the bourgeoisie (middle class), due to freedom of commerce, to the world market, to uniformity in the mode of production and in the conditions of life corresponding to growth. And yet Marx wanted to eliminate the middle class and private property. All those elements that were lowering the antagonisms between the lower and middle class was somehow not a consideration for honest capitalism.

6. *The Past*

Marx saw tradition as a tool of the (middle class). Observance to the past served as a mere distraction in proletariat's (working man) quest for emancipation and supremacy in his eyes.

In (middle class) society, Marx wrote, "the past dominates the present; in Communist society, the present dominates the past."

To paraphrase a statement, if we fail to look back at history (the past) we are doomed to repeat it. The danger of not looking back and seeing the pitfalls and the gains means we simply may fall to those pitfalls and overlook or never see the gains.

The influence of Carl Marx can been seen today in our society with the removing of Civil War monuments and statues by far leftists and BLM (Black Lives Matter). Marxism in principle is to tear down the norms that help stabilize the middle class and society has a whole.

We can see the attacks on enteral biological truths like 'man cannot become a woman or a woman cannot become a man,' moral devaluation, and pornography even within our elementary schools. This is where Communism abolishes moral truths and why it is now permeating our culture. Sense these action are not called communistic, no one recognizes what's taking place.

If unseen entities are influencing the elites that pull the strings of nations and states then their goal is to influence mankind in a way that would look appealing to them while lowering moral standards, putting them under greater control and eliminating individuality and independence. To get them to accept policies that would look like justice and right, while actually producing policies that would: Kill, steal and destroy an abundant future.

John 10:10-11

"The thief comes only to steal and kill and destroy. I came that they may have life and have it more abundantly."

It is the person of faith that will hold onto a promise and to recognize the pitfalls of policies that are simply godless in their principles.

Job 8:13: **"The same happens to all who forget God.**

The hopes of the godless evaporate."

Chapter 12

Evil Non-Human Entities Influencing the Mind of Man in History.

For those of us who believe there is a spiritual element to our existence, know this is the battle we fight.

A false prophet does not have to be a spiritual leader. He could be a governmental leader.

Matt 24:11

"And many false prophets shall arise, and shall lead many astray."

Top Ten Most Evil Dictators of All Time (in order of kill count) • Juan Carlos (readjuancarlos.com)

Most all the evil that has been perpetrated upon citizens of other nations in the past were either communists or authoritarian in principle.

These non-human entities have the capabilities to place ideas or even thoughts to manipulate the mind of man. It's like the downhill snowball effect. They plant the idea or thought and let man's nature take it from there.

Get the snowball rolling down-hill and it takes on a life of its own and grows bigger and bigger.

We often wonder when we look back in history how mankind could get to the point where they could commit such atrocities upon their fellow man.

We think those that do such horrific deed against men, women and children must have been monsters; that they are somehow just born that way? But that isn't always the case.

There is a documentary called *Ordinary Men*.

It was a documentary on World War 2 and how ordinary men became mass murderers.

There were some 60,000 men commissioned to round-up all the men, women and children that were Jewish and to take them to pits and shoot them, not to mention the gas chambers.

The men they commissioned were not killers, psychopath or homicidal maniacs. They were, plumbers, barbers, and carpenters from every field of Germany's working class. In many ways we would think these are the least likely men to become mass murders.

Most of these men were not eligible for regular military service due to their age and were put into the reservist part of the military.

In fact many weren't anti-Semites and they were of the age where they were not heavily influenced to the Nazification of Germany.

However there were other factors at work to motivate them that allowed them to commit such heinous acts upon the Jewish people.

Their commanders were not uneducated imbeciles. They were well educated and sophisticated and many could speak several different languages.

So what was it that made ordinary men commit mass murder?

When the soldiers were given the orders to commit such an act, they were also given the opportunity to back out and not follow the orders. They would receive no punishment from not following the order.

We would think, anyone given orders to kill innocent men, women and children would immediately back away or step out and refuse to comply with such a heinous order; no, only a very few refused to comply with the order to murder innocent men, women and children.

Those that did step out were not punished, but were rebuked and made fun of by their fellow soldiers. They called them sissy's, weak etc.

These men were not necessarily Nazis or the SS. They were ordinary men given orders by their government.

However we still haven't addressed just how these ordinary men could commit such evil acts and live with themselves?

Evil is not just a man-made construct. For those of us who believe in a creator and from a biblical perspective, we can see that God created man to have that internal moral compass.

Rom 2:14:

14 "Even Gentiles, who do not have God's written law, show that they know his law when they instinctively obey it, even without having heard it." LB

Yad Vashem wrote the book *Ordinary Men* and what he found focused upon the phycology of "group behavior."

It was: peer pressure, role adaptation, deference to authority in an atmosphere where there is no other support mechanism which shape the men's behavior in a group setting. Again, this points back to, "influence."

Things these men would do in a group setting that they would possibly never do as individuals.

On trial in the 1960s these men didn't give the normal excuse of, I was coerced or I had to do it or I would have been killed if I hadn't followed orders. They were all given the opportunity to not participate and not be punished for not following orders.

None of them could say, I had no choice because they all had a choice.

While it wasn't just one thing that motivated them to participate in the murder of men, women and children, (because everyone had their own reasons) it can be said that whatever excuse they gave, for everyone that did commit these heinous crimes, it was some kind of 'justification' in their minds that allowed them to follow through with this evil.

It was a group motivated act or we could say a mob mentality with each of them having different reason why they murdered innocent people.

Even when they committed the deed, many got sick and threw up and never wanted to participate again.

A justification that supplanted that internal God given moral code that says, this is wrong.

It is very much like the description of when Eve was presented to disobey God. There was a justification in

Eve's mind that allowed her to cross the line where God commanded her not to eat of the tree of knowledge. However her justification was inspired from an outside influence.

Once the men crossed that line, for whatever justification they had in their minds, to commit that act of murder, they now felt they were the victims.

As insane as that may sound to us, once a justification crosses that moral line, instead of having contrition, they make themselves the victim in defense of their heinous actions.

Wrong becomes right….and if not right, then the wrong was somehow justified because of someone else's fault, as a defense.

Chapter 13

Could Another Holocaust Be in the Future?

The word holocaust is a harsh word and gives us images of Nazi concentration camps and of the Jewish people being forced into railway cars heading to Auschwitz.

Some try and make a distinction between the words 'holocaust and genocide.' No matter how a person differentiates between the two words, both describes mass murders.

BBC Teach article listed here: The Holocaust year by year - BBC Teach

The article gives us a timeline of the Jewish holocaust. It shows that what took place was not an overnight or instant rounding up of the Jewish people but a slow burn. A gradual building up to where it finally escalated to the point where the powers that be, could carry out their heinous crimes of genocide.

It showed that the German government slowly conditioned the public to turn against the Jews to where they were looked upon as a problem to their society. They even looked upon the Jews as a virus.

1942 jews looked upon as a virus - Bing video

Throughout the 20th century there's been many genocides/holocausts. Communism alone is responsible for 100 million deaths.

Nov 6, 2017 Wall Street Journal

100 Years of Communism—and 100 Million Dead

The Bolshevik plague that began in Russia was the greatest catastrophe in human history
By David Satter.

Like: Nazism, Marxism and Communism, which display no conscience and can be dressed up many different way to accomplish their goals. I believe we are witnessing a dressed up form of Marxism/Communism here in the U.S. today in policies that have crippled our economy and methodically eliminating our middle class.

David Satter points out: "In a 1920 speech to the Komsomol, Lenin said that communists subordinate morality to the class struggle. Good was anything that destroyed "the old exploiting society" (they mean the middle class) and helped to build a "new communist society."

David Satter also says, This approach separated guilt from responsibility. Martyn Latsis, an official of the Cheka, Lenin's secret police, in a 1918 instruction to interrogators, wrote: "We are not waging war against individuals. We are exterminating the bourgeoisie (middle class) as a class. . . ."

What Are the Conditions for The Next Holocaust?

With every event where a genocide or holocaust has taken place it is almost AWAYS the government, a controlling military faction or the overtaking government that is behind the heinous acts against a certain segment of their population; whether politically, ethnically or religiously.

Could the next genocide come from the medical field on a global scale?

Division as a Tool?

During the Covid19 pandemic you had the American government segregate citizens into two groups. One group was considered compassionate and responsible. The other group was considered selfish, lacking compassion and ill-responsible. The other group of citizens were called by the American government, **"The Pandemic of The Unvaccinated."** The arm of the government, the mainstream press and social media platforms, jump on board and further fermented the notion that those who didn't take the vaccines were causing the deaths and hospitalizations.

It was, and still is, a partnership of private companies and government. Where the government could use the private sector to do their dirty work of enforcing compliance upon the America public and to publish misinformation and disinformation as factual to bring shame upon those who wouldn't follow the government direction.

You even had doctors and nurses who felt that those who were unvaccinated should not even have access to medical services. These sentiments were shocking. It was turning citizen against citizen. Very reminiscent of how the government turned its citizens against the Jewish people in Nazi Germany.

Dr. Robert Malone who is a virologist and early inventor of the mRNA process said in the article called Epoch Health Sept, 8th 2023: "This is one of the big lies that were spread, and it was weaponized to a point where we had a variety of key opinion leaders making ethically obscene statements, such as that people who would not take the vaccine should be denied medical care, hospitalization, the ability to participate in society; that they shouldn't be able to receive organ transplants. There was all of this jingoism-(fanaticism) promoted."

"Dr. Peter McCullough, an American cardiologist, called the COVID vaccines, 'the worst pharmaceutical development idea in the history of mankind.'"

"It often comes as a surprise to people that mRNA-type medical interventions and coronavirus vaccines had plenty of red flags through their history prior to December 2020. The ingredients used were already known to be toxic: Cationic lipids injure the nervous system, lungs and liver, as well as cell membranes throughout the body. Polyethylene glycol was never used for injections, due to safety concerns; mRNA had already been shown to change DNA. Previous attempts at coronavirus vaccines had all failed and killed the test animals. So inflicting the world's population with a new, mostly untested vaccine for which its components already had so many safety warnings was the most widespread reckless experiment in human history." --- Book review by Epoch Times - By Linda Wiegenfeld 9/20/23

Starting in 2020 the American government scared the public into such a frenzy that even if you didn't wear a mask, you were somehow a threat to the society.

I remember myself walking down a supermarket store isle … and I was going the wrong way because the arrow on the floor was pointing in the opposite direction. I had a mask on, but it was under my nose because I couldn't breathe well and I knew at that time, masks never stopped the virus.

The man who was heading my way had a mask on and on top of that he had a plastic face shield.

When he saw I was heading the wrong way and that I had my mask under my nose he started yelling at me. My response made him decide the best course of action was to walk on.

Much of our nation's response to Covid19 was in harmony with the WHO (World Health Organization) and the U.N.

Our NIH (National Institute of Health) and the CDC (Center for Disease Control) were in lockstep with the WHO and the U.N.

What our nation's mainstream news was failing to share with the public and even suppressing, what doctors from around the world were not only saying, that Covid19 is treatable but the vaccines are not only NOT stopping the virus, it was killing and injuring people at an unprecedented rate. And yet our CDC still continued to push a failed vaccine and boosters. Why would they do that?

Here is where we come to population control. Is it really just a conspiracy theory or is there evidence?

Many doctors and attorneys have the data and know there is something very wrong with what has taken place with Covid19 and the vaccines. Some are very fearful to say there is a de-population plan in motion, but their suspicion is, that is exactly what appears to be taking place.

As we mentioned earlier in our book, the WEF (World Economic Forum) believes we are over populated. They are working toward a one world governmental system where you will own nothing and be happy about not owning anything, according to them.

This very concept is a dressed up Communist solution for the world, but it's not called Communism and those who have no knowledge of history will not identify it.

They are masters at the psychology of using words that will make people feel good while losing their freedoms.

Anytime you see the words: Human Rights, Sustainable Development Goals, Fair and Equitable, Climate Action or Climate Change, 15 minute cities, Agenda 2030 etc., these are some of the dressed up words that cover for eliminating private property and bring in that one world governmental system that will control the population along with reducing the population.

In the article from Project Syndicate Sept. 10th 2019: GOTHENBURG/LONDON – On 2023 September 24-25, "world leaders will gather at the United Nations in New York to review progress toward the UN's 2030 Agenda and its 17 Sustainable Development Goals. The SDGs, which aim "to end poverty, protect the planet, and ensure prosperity for all," are commendable, and summarize the kind of world many of us wish to see in 2030. But if this vision is to have any chance of materializing, governments must now add an 18th goal: "Dampen population growth."

The BBC in 2011 says: "As the world reaches an estimated seven billion people, people like Vivek say efforts to bring down the world's population must continue if life on Earth is to be sustainable, and if poverty and even mass starvation are to be avoided."

It all sounds very reasonable, doesn't it?

Population control: Is it a tool of the rich? - BBC News

From the National Review titled, Population Implosion by Michael Brendon Dougherty March 29th 2021 writes: "Tyler Cowen writes about "global depopulation" as the looming existential threat no one is talking about."

Global Depopulation an Existential Threat | National Review

The idea of depopulation didn't start just a few years ago, it's been part of a global plan for many decades.

From the Frontline News, posted by Yudi Sherman December 24th 2023 "US Depopulation Hits New Milestone."

In the article it points out that the depopulation effort started decades ago and isn't just one tool to bring the population down but is multifaceted. Here is what some of that article said:

"Another of Jaffe's proposed actions was to place "fertility control agents in the water supply."

"Common pesticides have been found to not only dramatically effect fertility but to feminize males. In one study of the pesticide atrazine, most male frogs exposed to the toxin became attracted to other males. ... Most atrazine produced in the United States is manufactured by Syngenta, a company owned by the Chinese Communist Party."

The article also points out: "Another part of the strategy is using gender confusion ideology to prevent mass births. Whereas men and women naturally breed, masculinizing women and effeminizing men — contravening (meaning to violate) "gender norms" — is an effective way to stagnate a population."

"This may also explain why the US intelligence agencies are heavily funding gender confusion around the globe through "Pride" organizations and events."

Many have struggled to understand why the: gay, lesbian and transgender community are growing in such numbers. This helps to bring to light the possible reason why this is happening.

Then we have the "Club of Rome" which is comprised of high ranking politicians, scientists, businessmen and elites from 5 continents.

Their position is, even though there seems to be falling birthrates that alone won't solve the problem we face.

They believe the population may peak at 8.8. However to them the problem the world faces is not just population but consumption and over producing. Which also means they must find a way to lower the need for consumption and then in turn, producing needs will be reduced.

How that happens, we can only speculate that when you lower the population, eliminate capitalism (middle class) and all living needs are provided and monitored by a central (one world) government.

World 'population bomb' may never go off as feared, finds study | Population | The Guardian

There are many tools that the small group of unelected elites can use to depopulate without suspicion, such as: war, pandemics, pesticides, preservatives and often times telegraphing their intentions through social platforms and even through Hollywood movies. They do it in such a way that you don't suspect what their real goal is. Some call what Hollywood does by the name of "predictive programing."

With CIA assets imbedded in Hollywood they use the film industry to reveal what they plan to do in the future through their movies.

However there are others who are working toward this depopulation goal and using ways to convince us they care about saving people.

Bill Gates is urging governments around the world to prepare for future pandemics and smallpox terror attacks by investing billions in research and development. This would mean more vaccines for us, and possibly mandatory, which in turn means a lot more money for the vaccine companies and their investors.

Of course this brings us back to the issue of the Covid19 vaccines. We now believe that the vaccine saved no-one from getting the virus. In fact many doctors are reporting that you are more likely to get the Covid virus by taking the vaccine, which by all previous standards, is not a real vaccine.

Let's repeat this. We know from Barry Young the New Zealand whistle blower data release that possibly 13 – 17 million plus people have died from the vaccines worldwide and tens of millions injured. Thousands of those in New Zealand are believed to have died from the vaccines alone.

This was further validated by Barry Young statistic release:

"Mr. Young, a Ministry of Health employee-turned-whistleblower, examined connections between specific COVID-19 vaccine batches and mortality rates. What he found was alarming:

Batch ID 1: Total Vaccinated 711, Death Count 152, 21.38% Dead
Batch ID 8: Total Vaccinated 221, Death Count 38, 17.19% Dead
Batch ID 3: Total Vaccinated 310, Death Count 48, 15.48% Dead
Batch ID 4: Total Vaccinated 364, Death Count 37, 10.16% Dead
Batch ID 6: Total Vaccinated 1006, Death Count 101, 10.04% Dead

Batch ID 2: Total Vaccinated 1018, Death Count 98, 9.63% Dead

Batch ID 7: Total Vaccinated 38, Death Count 3, 7.89% Dead

Batch ID 72: Total Vaccinated 5882, Death Count 278, 4.73% Dead

Batch ID 62: Total Vaccinated 18173, Death Count 831, 4.57% Dead

Batch ID 71: Total Vaccinated 11019, Death Count 498, 4.52% Dead

The underlying mortality rate in New Zealand should be only 0.75%, said Young. So the odds of all these deaths happening by chance is approximately 100 billion to 1." (Meaning, deliberate).

"So statistically, what we're saying is that there is no chance that this vaccine is not a killer," declared Young."

As Naomi Wolf pointed out through the Pfizer documents, the 3rd adverse side effect from getting the vaccines is also getting infected with Covid.

We know money is involved with these vaccines that protect no one. However, we have to ask. Before Covid19 hit, the last time the CDC had pulled a vaccine off the market was when 56 people had died from the vaccine.

Something has changed because we now have some 30 thousand just in the U.S. who have died and 10s of thousands injured from these vaccines. That was the CDC VAERS report in early 2023 and only 1 percent of the reported cases; which means there is a possible 3 million alone in the U.S. that have died. That number I believe is growing.

However CDC-VAERS has changed things to where they have obfuscated the information on their web page.

So why haven't they pulled it from the market? Unless there is a goal besides money?

By August 2022, data analyst had compiled information on birth rate changes in 19 European countries and produced an extremely important paper. Nine months after the peak of COVID vaccinations, birth rates sharply declined and stayed down.

[Fourteen per cent decrease in live births in Europe nine months after the start of the COVID-19 pandemic and first lockdowns, researchers report | ScienceDaily](#)

Evidence, while antidotal at this time; cancers, aggressive cancers, have increased enormously since peak of the COVID vaccine in the spring of 2021.

There is no doubt that there is a nefarious agenda being played out. But who or what is influencing man with these ideas?

Invisible Battleground and The Non-Human Influence

Is man really being influenced by non-human entities as David Ike proposes and how the bible points out that there is a battle taking place in the invisible realm?

For many who may hear of these depopulation scenarios find it incomprehensible or simply unbelievable. Who would do such a thing?

But again, who would take innocent: men, women and children and slaughter them like they did in Nazi Germany?

The incomprehensible or even the unbelievable is often a cover to accomplish that which people cannot believe would happen.

Chapter 14

Consciousness and The Non-Human Connection

Our world is more connected in unimaginable ways than most people realize.

Many may have never heard of Ben Rich. Ben Rich was the head of Lockheed Martin's, Skunk Works, which is the official pseudonym for Lockheed Martin's "Advance Development Programs."

It is a highly classified research company that is responsible for: the U-2 Spy plane, SR71 Blackbird, F-117 Nighthawk, F-22 Raptor, and the F-35 Lighting ll.

Ben Rich retired from Skunk Works in 1991. He gave his last talk to a body of people:

"We already have the means to travel among the stars but these technologies are locked up in Black Projects... and it would take an act of God to ever get them out to benefit humanity. Anything you can imagine, we already know how to do."

He also said: "We now have the technology to take ET home. No, it won't take someone's lifetime to do it. There is an error in the equations. We know what it is. We now have the capability to travel to the stars."

– Ben Rich, Former Director of Lockheed Skunk works shortly before his passing. -

"Ben Rich was asked how UFO propulsion functioned. His reply was revealing. He replied to the man asking the question, "Let me ask you. How does ESP work?" The man asking the question of Mr. Rich said – "All points in time and space are connected?" Ben Rich then replied, "That's how it works!"

There was more than one confirmation of Ben Rich's words on the subject of UFOs. Here is one:

William Hamilton wrote, "Rich Andrews was a close personal friend of Lockheed's "Skunk Works" CEO Ben Rich, the hand-picked successor of Skunk Works founder Kelly Johnson and the man famous for the F-117 Nighthawk "Stealth" fighter, its prototype the HAVE BLUE. Before Rich died of cancer, Andrews took my questions to him. Rich confirmed:

There are two types of UFOs — the ones we build, and ones THEY build. We learned from both crash retrievals and actual "Hand-me-downs." The Government knew, and until 1969 took an active hand in the administration of that information. After a 1969 Nixon "Purge", administration was handled by an international board of directors in the private sector." --- NEXUS Newsfeed.com.

Think about this. When Ben Rich was asked how UFO's work, his response was with a question. How does ESP work? The man answered by saying, 'All points in time and space are connected?' Ben Rich said, that is how it works.

What that means is, consciousness. That thought is faster than the speed of light. It is the ability to move the craft through space-time where there is no inertia experienced.

This is why they say you can see the UFO move at extreme speeds make a 90 degree turn without slowing down. There is no sonic boom when flying faster than the speed of sound because, even though you can see them, they are just outside our space-time. It also means they can travel great distances in a very short time. Something beyond our reported capabilities.

As an example. Alpha Centauri is the nearest star system to the Sun, located at the distance of 4.37 light years away. That means we would have to travel at 186 thousand miles per-second for over 4 years to reach Alpha Centauri. That is approximately 25.8 trillion miles from us.

However, to travel at the speed of thought supersedes all our known laws of physics. Traveling at the speed of thought covers distance unachievable by light speed within a person's life span. At the speed of thought it would be a matter of seconds or a few minutes to reach Alpha Centauri.

It is consciousness and how things are connected. Which brings us back to mankind being influenced through his mind or consciousness.

Dr. Steven Greer.

Dr. Steven Greer is the head of the CE5 or CSETI (Center for the Study of Extraterrestrial Intelligence and the Disclosure Project).

I had mentioned earlier that David Crusch and Tom DeLonge had a position in common. But now Dr. Steven Greer, Tom DeLonge, David Crusch, Ben Rich and even the famed Bob Lazar of area 51 all have something in common.

They have all said, these beings or crafts we call UFO's, function on or through, "consciousness."

Dr. Karla Turner

There is one person that is seldom mentioned when it comes to UFO's and alien contact.

Dr. Karla Turner was respected in the UFO community and had accomplished serious and credible research in the field. She passed away in 1996 from breast cancer.

Dr. Turner was a human rights activist and she believed she had been abducted and from that experience became an alien abduction investigator.

She had a background in Old English Studies and was a former college instructor, she authored three books on the abduction phenomenon: Into the Fringe (1992), Taken (1994), and Masquerade of Angels (1994), co-written with psychic Ted Rice. Her work in this area raised grave questions about the actual nature and intentions of these extraterrestrial encounters.

Dr. Tuner didn't come from a spiritual or Christian perspective but rather just solid research and data approach.

Dr. Karla Turner spent time in studying alien abduction accounts since around 1988. In her books "Into the Fringe" and "Taken," she shared her abduction experiences and the stories of other abductees, emphasizing the disturbing events that transpired.

Unlike Dr. Steven Greer who believes non-human entities (extraterrestrials) are mostly all good and are here to help humanity. Dr. Tuner had a very different experience in the opposite direction.

In "Masquerade of Angels," she described the experiences of Ted Rice, (a physic) who relied upon his spirit guide for many years. He slowly come to realize that his spirit guide wasn't who he thought. He later found that there was a UFO connection. He initially believed his spirit guide to be of a benevolent nature; later came to realize their predatory and destructive nature.

That was many years down the line. His spirit guide had helped him and others, which initially made him believe they were a benevolent guide.

(Remember, evil spirits can do good, but for nefarious purposes).

One particular account involved Ted Rice as an 8-year-old boy, witnessing his deceased grandfather transforming into a reptilian type being and demanding intimacy with him. The sexual encounter by these entities is something that is recorded in history that I'll address a little later.

I agree with Dr. Karla Turner that they have the ability to manipulate perception. What I would like to point out, if they can manipulate how we perceive things individually, then they can also manipulate world leaders and how they view what our future should look like?

Tom DeLonge and now others, who are working closely with the government, point out these "others" use <u>mankind like chest pieces.</u> They create conflicts and war. Warfare is one way of manipulating man and thinning the population without suspicion.

A great deal of information has made its way to the public or available to the public through whistle blowers and experiencers.

Much of what is shared in this book is not found in mainstream news or mainstream social media platforms. However it is out there and it only takes a person to spend the time researching.

Most don't have the time to spend hours reading and researching and to access the information from those who do the footwork in order to reveal to the public just what is taking place, which the mainstream refuse to cover.

Vicky Verma wrote in the "How&Why" 2023/05/19 article speaking of Dr. Turner:

Before her death, she frequently spoke at UFO conferences in the United States and other countries, urging people to take action. She claimed that aliens were manipulating our perceptions and spreading disinformation to weaken us and deceive us into thinking they cared about us, when in reality, their intentions were self-serving and disregarded our well-being. Turner emphasized the need to regain control over the situation and confront these aliens. Dr. Turner discovered these seven basic elements of the alien abduction phenomenon published by John Chambers in the UFO Magazine

I'm going to list some of the things she found and they will sound very bazaar and unbelievable, especially for those who have little to no knowledge concerning this topic. The people she interviewed were not crazy or had struggle with mental illness prior to the encounters.

1. Aliens can control what we think we see. They can appear to us in any number of guises and shapes; **(This fits in with the book of Enoch where he points out that spirits reveal themselves in many different forms and deceive mankind).**

2. Aliens can take us – our consciousness – out of our physical bodies, disable our control of our bodies, install one of their own entities, and use our bodies as vehicles for their own activities before returning our consciousness to our bodies; **(This can also be looked at as a possible possession or where people can't move at night but are awake and something preventing movement).**

3. Aliens can be present with us in an invisible state and can make themselves only partially visible; **(Again, this can fall under ghosts and poltergeists).**

4. A surprising number of abductees suffer from serious illnesses they didn't have before their encounters. These have led to surgery, debilitation, and even death from causes the doctors can't identify.

5. Some abductees experience a degeneration of their mental, social and spiritual well-being. Excessive behavior frequently erupts, such as drug abuse, alcoholism, overeating and promiscuity. Strange obsessions develop and cause the disruption of normal life and the destruction of personal relationships. **(This can fall under spiritual oppression or some may call it demonic oppression).**

These experiences or events listed here can be found throughout-history. Starting in the Garden of Eden mankind has been manipulated and influenced in one way or another.

Dr. Karla Turner was asked by a lady on the radio with Art Bell's Dream Land show, what she thought the bible meant when they refer to demons.

Dr. Turner responded by saying that the bible could be referring to these type of beings. She didn't know for sure.

Dr. Turner states that with abductions there can be cures along with harming. There doesn't appear to be just one direction of healing or harming, but rather both cures and harming come with the abduction scenario.

Let me point out that author Heather Lynn, PhD who wrote on the history of evil spirits called "Evil Archaeology" that evil spirits could do both good and evil. Often the good was for deceptive purposes.

As I pointed out in my second book *"Blindsided, UFO's, Government and God"* the gods of mythology did good and evil and influenced kings and kingdoms. Which means our world governments are vulnerable to the manipulation by non-human influence.

Chapter 15

UFO and Religious Experience?

According to Dr. Karla Turner, there is a vast range of events connected to the UFO and alien abduction scenario that she felt no one seem to be able to put a finger on and say it's just this or just that.

These events appears to have the secular UFO researcher confused or baffled about just who these beings are and their purpose here.

Karla Turner Claimed She Found Evidence That Aliens Are Manipulating Human Reality (howandwhys.com)

Tom DeLonge in his early interviews and also one in 2023 mentioned that when he was briefed or read-in on the "Others" or extraterrestrials, he was so disturbed and shaken by what he found out that he could not sleep for 3 days.

In interviews he had been asked repeatedly, what was it that kept you up for 3 day? He would never come right out and say just what it was that disturbed him so badly that he couldn't sleep.

In like manor the rumors of President Jimmy Carter when finally being read-in on extraterrestrials was said to have placed his head in his hands and proceeded to cry. He was noticeably disturbed for weeks after.

Tom DeLonge also pointed out that when information on who and what these beings are gets exposed or revealed it will shake the religious world to its core. He is hoping that religion won't crumble but adapt to the new revelation.

What does that really mean, to adapt to that new revelation? Because from what is being espoused from those in the know (government sources), all religions were created by them.

Is man then going to look to them and worship these beings?

There is no doubt many who have had a close UFO encounter have some kind of a spiritual or religious experience or component to it.

Dr. Jacques Vallée a computer scientist and one of the most credible UFO researchers, believes that when investigating a UFO encounter, the focus should be on the witness, how he or she interpreted the event, and how it affected their life (he noted that many people tend to emotionally react to a UFO sighting as a spiritual or religious experience).

Mind Manipulation and Perception

Having come this far in the examination of *The Invisible Battleground and Non-Human Influence* and of UFOs and mind manipulation, this invisible spiritual battle reveals a connection in scripture, including the work of many good secular researchers.

I strongly believe the entities that secular UFO researchers say are alien or dimensional beings from another world or dimension, are in fact the very beings that Jehovah God created. "They are one in the same."

Vicky Verma – 03/13/2023, wrote an article about Jeremey Corbell the documentary filmmaker. Corbell does an excellent job in laying out the struggles behind those who claim to have personal knowledge of UFO's.

In the article it reveals that he, along with George Kapp, has had contact and possibly inside information from those who may deal directly with this topic. It has given Corbell a direction of what may really be taking place. Here is a sample of his statement:

"UFOs appear to be part of a larger phenomenon meaning UFOs are kind of an auxiliary implication of a much larger reality. So this idea that what we're seeing are machines from other planets. I'm unconvinced what we may be seeing is an alternate reality. You know maybe it is something closer to dimensional travel.

There seems to be another version of reality that is occurring and that somehow once they pop through into our reality. And this is not just from a cursory look at the UFO phenomenon, this is from talking with thousands of close encounter eyewitnesses who tell me that this is something bigger than just flying machines.

To give you an example at Skinwalker Ranch. The report is that a piece of the sky opened up like a tear and out of this came "Beings" came "Craft." So, UFOs is a symptom, its part of this alternate reality, the phenomenon as I call it. But it's not just about UFOs that represent this phenomenon."

It's often inconceivable for the average person or the secular UFO researcher to see how the UFO/Alien phenomenon could be fallen angels or beings that Jehovah God created. However scripture is replete with examples of beings who somehow move in and out of our dimension.

People (Christian & Secular) tend to look at scripture in the framework of Roman soldiers and horse drawn carts.

Biblical scriptures the book of Enoch and other writings around the world reveal that these spirits/entities can appear in many different forms. It also means they have a certain ability that we can't hardly conceive of.

Our United States government calls them the "*Others*" and not aliens. They consider them god like and do not believe they are fully benevolent. In fact from what Tom DeLonge has revealed and others, our government, those in the know, are scared.

This means there is a part of our government that has had and may still be in contact with these non-human entities.

They have the ability to manipulate the mind of mankind. To manipulate perceptions and to induce hate and anger. This is one reason why Tom DeLonge and others believe we must focus on love. To set our vibrational energy on a higher plain.

<u>However, to do that without the creator of love becomes a deception.</u>

There are two forces at odds with each other. 1. There is a false love from the god of this world.

2 Cor 11:14-15

14 And no wonder, for even Satan disguises himself as an angel of light.

2 Cor 4:4-5:

"In their case the god of this world has blinded the minds of the unbelievers, to keep them from seeing the light of the gospel of the glory of Christ, who is the image of God." ESV

The god of this worlds goal is to destroy faith or if not destroy it completely, to remove any direction that would lead to a faith in Christ.

2. God who created all things and is revealed in Jesus the son.

John 14:6-7

"Jesus told him, "I am the way, the truth, and the life. No one can come to the Father except through me."

1 John 4:8-11

"Anyone who does not love does not know God, because God is love. 9 In this the love of God was made manifest among us, that God sent his only Son into the world, so that we might live through him. 10 In this is love, not that we have loved God but that he loved us and sent his Son to be the propitiation (paid the price) for our sins." ESV

This is the battle of the two powers. As old fashion as it may sound. The devil that the church has described over the years to the believers has been very limited and lacking in who the adversary really is and the capabilities of deception they possess.

The believers must open their eyes to adversary capabilities.

In the story of Daniel he had humbled himself and God heard his prayer and sent an angel to let him know that his prayer was heard but had to have help from Michael the arch-angel because he was held back for 20 days by the adversary. Dan. 10:12-14.

These entities by virtue of their very nature have the ability to produce: technologies, become physical or in spirit form, can appear as many different races of alien beings. They have over eons given mankind the ability to advance technologically, agriculturally and culturally. As both George Knapp and Tom DeLonge has made the claim, they also have the ability to manipulate mankind into wars.

We have the Ukraine war with Russia at the time of this writing. We have China in preparation to take over Taiwan. At this writing we have Hamas that have attacked Israelis with the slaughter of innocent men, women and children. People blaming each side and causing unrest.

The possibility of a 3rd world war is closer than ever before. It is a real possibility.

We often don't realize how we can be manipulated, even when we think we know what's going on.

Tom DeLonge's media endeavors

Tom DeLonge's goal is to reach the youth of our nation and of the world. With a message that God is not some guy in long robes walking around in Birkenstock shoes.

In other words, don't look to Jesus because he's just another alien being or avatar.

He believes that Christianity, Muslim, Atheist etc. just keep you blocked in to what is really out there.

The movie that Tom DeLonge produced, *Monsters of California,* is done very well. While it does have a lot of harsh language in it, it's entertaining, funny and directed more toward the younger generation.

The average person that watches it will not pick up on the connection that much of what he has in the movie reflects his relationship with his mother in real life and the possible connection to his father and how he was able to get involved with the government on such a deep level.

It reveals that our government, who has lied to the American public for some 80 plus years, does know about entities they considers god-like and are scared by their capabilities.

This information, no doubt, has to challenge the minds of many people; to think that there really are alien type beings with god-like powers and has been influencing mankind from the beginning and that our government has known about this for decades. This will undoubtedly be unsettling and frighten many.

The government whistle blower, David Crusch reveals that our government has been working many years to back engineer crashed or captured non-human vehicles.

Tom DeLonge's movie is not only a conditioning to get people to think about not being alone in our universe. I also believe this is a government sponsored or government sanctioned process of a slow controlled disclosure to the public about the reality of these entities.

A large portion of our government knows very little to nothing about this issue. It is highly secure and secret part of our government that is working toward a controlled disclosure. However it is an enteral battle because there are factions that don't want this to be revealed.

For many, *Monsters of California* movie will make sense, especially for those who have no spiritual or biblical foundation, and will convey a message that Jesus is only one of many god like beings. That all the religions can possibly become one. Very much the way that we might think of as a one world religion; if religion is even going to be around after this becomes openly known.

Religion may be around but will true faith?

Luke 18:8:

Nevertheless when the Son of man returns, shall he find faith on the earth?

What will be the challenge to those of faith if and when it becomes known that non-human beings are responsible for all the religions in our world?

Chapter 16

Why Hasn't the News That UFO's & Alien Beings Are Real, Captured World Headlines?

On May 9, 2001, some twenty military, intelligence, government, corporate and scientific witnesses came forward to share their first-hand experience at the National Press Club in Washington, DC to corroborate the reality of UFOs or what some call extraterrestrial vehicles, extraterrestrial life forms, and advanced energy and propulsion technologies. Credible and distinguished witnesses that should have garnered, if not worldwide, at least national attention.

Then some 20 years later on July, 27th 2023 we had three military veterans testify in Congress' on UFO's, including a former Air Force intelligence officer who claimed the U.S. government has operated a secret "multi-decade" reverse engineering program of recovered vehicles. He also said the U.S. has recovered non-human "biologics" from alleged crash sites. That was Major David Charles Crusch.

Then again in 2023 the Twitter file author Michael Shellenberger was interviewed by "The Hill Rising" stated high ranking officials have come out in support saying what David Crusch has claimed is real and verifiable.

Also that our military and non-human entities have had some kind of interaction.

Shellenberger said there was information that he received that he deliberately kept out of his report because it was just too shocking.

I would loved to have that information. I may not have wrote about it or revealed it either. Because, even if it is real and verifiable, if it is too extreme, people will not believe it and discard anything you may share.

(2) 12 ALIEN CRAFT In US Custody, Per Intel: Michael Shellenberger; Single Source Claims PILOT Recovered - YouTube

So why has the news that UFO's and non-human entities are real, not dominated world headlines?

To answer that question we have to look back at over 70 years of a psychological disinformation and misinformation program by the United States government to shame, ridicule and besmirch anyone who would claim to have had a sighting or had contact.

As Edgar Mitchell, the fourth man to walk on the moon said, the information has been getting out there but it's been a misinformation and disinformation program by our government. It's been hiding in plain sight.

So the public, through the conditioning by our government, still has either disbelief or fear to believe that UFO's and non-human entities are real. The fear of ridicule pushes people to continue to believe it's all make believe.

Our government has built a psychological brick wall that must now be knocked down.

However, government and former government leakers are coming forward. In a Newsbreak article:

Aliens will "reveal themselves" in 2027 claims ex-CIA agent

By Bernadette Giacomazzo & John O'sullivan, 11/14/2023

"A former CIA agent says that aliens will reveal themselves to humanity in four years' time, reports The Express . John Ramirez, who has extensive experience working with the United States governmental agency, told Podcast UFO that extraterrestrials - after all the talk of governmental cover-ups and alien discoveries - are keen to introduce themselves to humans."

Whether this is a false flag or not, this coming reveal has been in the planning for many years. The article goes further to state:

"We're kind of preparing the U.S. population at least, and by extension the world population, to that reality," 'the former agent said.' "That there is a presence here and that we need to explain this presence. Because if they show up and we continue to do what we did before in previous decades, there will be mass panic."

As I mentioned in my first and second books this is the third paradigm shift in mankind's consciousness about who we are and where we came from.

It is that third paradigm shift that is the greatest deception in human history. That we were created by these aliens. That Jesus/Jehovah God is only one of many non-human entities or avatars that are responsible for all the religions upon this earth. They are the mythological gods of antiquities.

With all the political wrangling's and waring of nations, preparation in the condition of man's thought and belief process has been shaping up for a worldwide massive deception.

In 2016 before I released my first book I was saying that more and more would be coming out and revealed on this topic of UFOs. So far this has been the case.

These alien beings are in fact the fallen angles and disembodied spirits of the bible. They are the dimensional beings of the UFO phenomenon and many secular researchers are coming to the position that they aren't beings from another planet but seem to be dimensional or what some call interdimensional.

From the article "How&Why" by Vicky Verma 2022/09/22:

"American journalist John Keel (1930-2009) was a believer in extraterrestrials and speculated that the stories from folklore and religious texts were proof that humanity had indeed made contact with another form of intelligent life, but that they were not from outer space. Instead, they were beings from other dimensions: ultraterrestrials

Keel theorized that those beings could shapeshift to look like anything, and attributed them to stories of demons, monsters, angels, ogres and changelings. He thought those ultraterrestrials likely had a sense of right and wrong, and that they were capable of manipulating mankind.

One of the benefits of the Interdimensional Hypothesis according to Hilary Evans (1929-2011), a British pictorial archivist, author, and researcher into UFOs and other paranormal phenomena, is that it can explain the apparent ability of UFOs to appear and disappear not only from sight but from radar; as the interdimensional UFO's can enter and leave our dimension at will, meaning they have the ability to materialize and dematerialize."

Yet there has been so much revealed to the public through articles, television broadcasts etc., and still nothing has captured the world's attention.

That time is coming. However the affect that it brings with the revelations of non- human entities has been in the planning for many decades.

Chapter 17

Decades of Deceptive Planning

We often think what we're experiencing in our world today is just a matter of bad planning or people who have a different point of view on how to run things. We only wish that was true. It's a lot more nefarious than that.

Before Edward Snowden and Julian Assange there was a man by the name of William Cooper. He was a former Naval Intelligence briefing team member.

What he learned during those years in the intelligence field, he made the choice, like Snowden, to come out and reveal secret government files that were kept since the 1940s. He was a patriot.

These are not the files that just reveal a plot against adversarial governments, although that was a part of it. No, these files were plots against an American president and the American public, by our government.

From the information he acquired was able to predict the fall of the Berlin Wall, and the invasion of Panama. All his predictions took place before those events occurred.

William Cooper had compiled documents that reveal a staggering scenario of corruption by our government. His book, filled with documentation, is called *"Behold A Pale Horse."*

He had endorsements:

"Bill Cooper is the world's leading expert on UFOs."
–Billy Goodman, KVEG, Las Vegas

"The only man in America who has all the pieces to the puzzle that has troubled so many for so long." – Anthony Hilder, Radio Free America

"William Cooper may be one of America's greatest heroes, and this story may be the biggest story in the history of the world." -Mills Crenshaw, KALK, Salt Lake City

Much of what he reveals was never reported in the mainstream press simply because the press is controlled by the elites who control America's corporate media platforms.

William Cooper points out in his book:

"On the day I learned that the office of Naval Intelligence had participated in the assassination of President John

F. Kennedy and that it was the Secret Service agent driving the limo that had shot Kennedy in the head, I went AWOL with no intention of ever returning. My good friend Bob Swan is the one who talked me into going back. Later, on June 1, 1972, the eve of my wedding, I told Bob everything that I knew about the UFOs; Kennedy's assassination; the Navy; the Secret Government; the coming ice age; Alternatives 1, 2, and 3; Project Galileo; and the plan for the new world order. I believed it was all true then, and I believe it's all true now.

I must warn you however, that I have found evidence that the secret societies were planning as far back as 1917 to invent an artificial threat from outer space in order to bring humanity together in a one-world government that they call the New World Order. I'm still searching for the truth. I firmly believe that this book is closer to that truth than anything ever previously written."

If you can find this on YouTube, his lecture will reveal even more than I do here.

William Cooper alternetive 1, 2 and 3 at DuckDuckGo

To be clear, I have seen a video clip of the limo driver leaning back with his arm extended toward JFK. I could not tell if he had a gun or shoot due to the graininess of the clip. Many believe this to be false about the limo driver. However that video clip is nowhere to be found, as it has disappeared.

We do know however for a fact, our government was involved in the JFK assassination.

William Cooper had several attempts on his life and eventually they accomplished their goal and was shot and killed in 2001 before getting this book out. From what I understand it was those close to him that worked to publish his book for him.

Some might say, what he describes in his book are just the plans of evil men, and that would be true. However, these evil plans come from the dark regions of the mind that is influenced by non-human entities. You may scoff at that, many do.

Years ago the comedy act of Flip Wilson use to say, "The Devil made me do it." While that was funny and garnered many laughs. The reality is, the devil didn't make people do these things that harm humanity, but these adversarial spirit/beings (some call demons) influenced them through their minds. In like manor the elites and heads of states become convinced that their plans are for the betterment of humanity and work to convince the population in a covert way and hide the nefarious action they take to accomplish their goals.

Void from the belief in God the creator who is represented in the person of Jesus, opens these world leaders to the influence of these entities that are at war with the creator. They are convinced in their minds that what they are imposing on humanity is best for the future.

The goal is to eradicate humanity as we know it. To change what it means to be human.

For us, when we look back we can see the psychological conditioning along with the biological manipulation or tampering of DNA along with the cultural grooming and the educational indoctrination that has been taking place for decades. All this is in the preparation to bring about a one world government and a post-human, as God created, future.

The constant bombardment and abuse in conditioning us to shape the direction for a post-human future is not what many can wrap their minds around. Mankind is being manipulated psychosocially to accept what is un-natural, as natural and irrational as rational in almost every fascist human interaction.

The future mankind faces, some like to call a hyper-controlled Matrix. It is a future where the population is reduced, controlled and alter what it means to be human. It is a trans-human world they are working for. It is the extinction of the God created human-race.

The unseen influence works through the elites of our world to control mankind's perception of reality.

Traditional standards of morality in society and governance must be tore down. Their methods are to: Destabilize, Dehumanize and Demoralize through all possible means.

As we mentioned concerning Marxism/Communism which they repackage those principles for a more modern age. It starts with the destruction of the nuclear family, the elimination of private property, and creating dependency upon government. Control our children's indoctrination by the public school system, ran by the state, along with abortion and the elimination of God to change the mindset of who we are and where we come from.

In every possible or conceivable way mankind is being attacked in a way that has been incremental to where they can now openly be more blatant about their goals and approaches to implementations.

William Cooper pointed out that America is in a state of apathy and are being led like sheep to the slaughter.

That was never more evident than when we were subjected to the Covid19 lockdowns, masking and required vaccines that have now been proven to be deadly. Yet our media and the government continue to push this deadly concoction.

It's not just America. It's the world.

Chapter 18

Our Strange Reality

Rev 16:12-16

13 And I saw three evil spirits that looked like frogs leap from the mouths of the dragon, the beast, and the false prophet. 14 <u>They are demonic spirits who work miracles and go out to all the rulers of the world to gather them for battle against the Lord on that great judgment day of God the Almighty.</u>

Mark Twain once said: "Truth is stranger than fiction, because fiction has to make sense, truth doesn't."

We must always remember that the book of Revelations is highly symbolic and not represented as literal but rather symbolizing a connection or representative of events or actions taken or to come.

So let's focus for now on the areas of the: "dragon, beast and false prophet." The three spirits of deception.

1. The Dragon. The Greek word for dragon is "Drakon or Drassomai" and can be defined as: a fabulous serpent, capturing, grasp or to entrap.

This spirit (dragon) is very shrewd, wise, strategic and cunning. It means that this spirit works to capture and entrap mankind through deception, using all possible tools to entrap the mind and belief of mankind. This has been the work of this spirit from the Garden of Eden.

Jesus even used the illustration of a serpent as being wise and strategic but tells his followers to be harmless:

Matt 10:16

"Behold, I send you out as sheep in the midst of wolves. Therefore be wise as serpents and harmless as doves. NKJV

2. The Beast. Comes from two Greek words:2342-Theerion and 2344 Theesauros-Theesaurou and deals with a store house, treasury which valuables are kept and repository.

In looking at biblical prophecy the beast, like in the book of Daniel and Revelations, most often is represented as man's system, nations or government. Man's system of government is a repository that holds its citizens taxes.

Throughout history, the system of man (governments) often start out as somewhat beneficial to man, and end up either collapsing and throwing its citizens into despair due to corruption or enslaving their citizens. This is that Mark of the Beast (man's system of government) where it will eventually control humanity through technology.

3. The False Prophet. From the Greek word: NT:5578 pseudoprofeetees, pseudoprofeetou, ho one who, acting the part of a divinely inspired prophet, or utters falsehoods under the name of divine prophecies, a false prophet. One who speaks of the future as a vision of what should or will be.

This represents religion that can also be a part of a government and the religious world.

Islam is not only a religion but a governmental system. The Vatican is religious and also a government and considered the smallest nation on earth.

Keep in mind that falsehoods, appear as truth, utterly convincing to the hearer. This happens even within the Christian community of false teachers and prophets. Matt. 7:21-23

These three spirits are spirits of deception with each of the Dragon, Beast and False Prophet.

What are the characteristic of the "frogs" that jumped out of the Dragon, Beast and False Prophet?

The answer is, they catch their prey with their tongue.

These three spirits are the three spirits that are responsible for the three paradigm shifts in man's consciousness and to change the mindset of who we are and where we come from.

1. From the gods who gave man knowledge, technology, agriculture and then became the gods of mythology.
2. Then angels and demons. Within the angel and demon period there was an explosion of superstition.
3. The final deception of angels and demons to be viewed as UFO/aliens of other races of beings and who created all the religions of the world and created mankind.

It is a long term plan of deception being played out in our world today.

The gods of antiquities that set up governments and give technologies to advance mankind were the gods that Jehovah God reprimanded for allowing wickedness to increase.

Repeating this verse.

Ps 82:1-2

"God has taken his place in the divine council; in the midst of the "gods" he holds judgment: 2 "How long will you judge unjustly and show partiality to the wicked?" ESV

Capable Deception

What are the capabilities of the entities behind the UFO phenomenon?

Here is what I found and what I believe due to what I have discovered from past and present researchers. It is a culmination of data that brings me to this position.

These entities that people see as UFO's and (Christian religion calls demons) are spiritual/dimensional beings. While some may see them as an alien race of beings from a far off galaxy or ultra-dimensional, they do not come from another planet or universe; although they are capable of traversing the expanse of space.

Jude 6 **"And I remind you of the angels who did not stay within the limits of authority God gave them but left the place where they belonged."**

These beings are the creation of who the Jew's call, Jehovah and the Christians believe Jehovah is represented in the person of Jesus. He is that one source of all creation. His creation rebelled and became the lords and gods of many cultures and religions upon earth.

1 Cor 8:5-7 **"For though there be that are called gods, whether in heaven or on earth; as there are gods many, and lords many; 6 yet to us there is one God, the Father, of whom are all things, and we unto him; and one Lord, Jesus Christ, through whom are**

all things, and we through him. 7 Howbeit there is not in all men that knowledge:" ASV

The secular world sees them as aliens and even having a spiritual element to them. Yet the secular researcher or investigator will reject any connection that they are related to the Christian Judeo bible, and if they do connect it, it is only to say, these are really aliens and not demons or what God created.

The secular world sees their abilities as a form of advanced technologies. And in many ways they are advanced technologically. However, their abilities come from their very nature which can appear and even produce a form of technology.

They are capable of appearing in any form as a means of deception. That means they can appear as many different alien races or as a loved one who has passed on. They have the ability of materializing solid material which can include technologies, organic properties, whether in a physical form or apparitions. There is a pattern that connects: ghosts, poltergeists, shadow people, paranormal apparitions, mediums, remote viewing, cryptoid-creatures, beings of light, Orbs, crop-circles and of course, UFOs, that all indicate a single sources.

They can know your thoughts because they operate on a certain level of vibration and consciousness. They can plant thoughts into mankind as a means to manipulate through emotion and feelings. This is why many are fooled to believe there are many different race of beings out there. Some for our good while others for the bad of mankind. They operate on a level of consciousness and frequency.

UFO crashes where there were recovered technologies and dead bodies or sightings that has taken place, is because they planned it or allowed it. Some of the crashes were planned centuries ago. The technologies they allowed us to recover have been dumbed down for us, yet so far beyond what we can sometime imagine.

Their actual abilities to operate and function and to manipulate time and space is so far beyond the technologies that we have thus far recovered and now use (although, I'm beginning to suspect that we are at times manipulating time and space.) Their abilities to produce what we consider technologies again, comes from their very nature.

However it is our own minds that they are capable of using against us. Jacques Vallee, the famed computer scientist and also portrayed in the Steven Spielberg movie "Close Encounters of the Third Kind" as the lead scientist is an agnostic, believes in real life that these entities have been, over many centuries, manipulating the minds of humans.

Dr. Jacque Vallee, Dr. David Jacob's and Dr. Karla Turner all point to the manipulation of the mind. Their assertion validates scripture that says, "We are not ignorant to Satan's device." Again, this word "device" in scripture, represents our minds.

Whether people realize it or not, the world is being used by these entities and influenced through the manipulation of the mind; and have been from the beginning of our human birth.

Tom DeLonge says that our government knows of these beings and have been preparing for a possible conflict with these beings in the future. Also that some of our technology comes from these beings through the process of reverse engineering.

The connection of where these entities come from are often overlooked by other secular researchers even though a fellow secular researcher may reveal that there might be a biblical connection. Dr. Jacque Vallee who has authored a number of books points this out:

"Messengers of Deception:" "The UFO phenomenon and the occupants is strikingly similar to that which is connected to demons." He also writes in his book called "Confrontations." "The medical examinations to which abductions are said to be subjected, often accompanied by sadistic sexual manipulation, is reminiscent of medieval tales of encounters with demons."

Dr. Jacque Vallee, Dr. David Jacob's and Dr. Karla Turner all point to the manipulation of the mind. Let me say this again, their assertion validates scripture that says, "We are not ignorant to Satan's device." It is our minds they are able to influence."

Let me share another section from of my book "Out Of The Box Faith."

1. "Karla Turner PhD and author of "Into the Fringe, Taken and also Masquerade of Angels" claims she and her husband are abductees. Before she passed away in 1996 she said that these entities are not what people think they are. Many have been tricked or deceived into believing that some or all of them are benevolent. Some believe they are here to help mankind save our planet. However Dr. Turner and Dr. David Jacobs along with Dr. Jacque Vallee, believe this is a deception. According to Dr. Turner and others, they can appear to you in many different forms. Her claim is the same as that of Tom DeLonge's statement; they deceive and lie.
2. Many people, who are researchers and experiencers, believe the grays and reptoids are among many other races of aliens. Given Dr. Turner's statement that they can appear to be something they aren't and that they lie and are untrustworthy, is consistent with Tom DeLonge's statement that they are not truthful beings.

Dr. Turner believes that these entities deliberately deceive us. For what reason, she didn't know. She says they are masters at the illusionary experience. They can make us believe or see anything they want and it is as real as reality itself."

This no doubt may all sound strange and even unbelievable to the reader. However consider that ancient tribes in the Amazon that have not experienced our technologies being told we have the ability to talk to people around the world instantaneously or see them on the other side of the world. It would be un-comprehendible to them. They wouldn't be able to wrap their minds around how that would even work.

Consider this. Those people in the Amazon are thousands of years behind us. They have not progressed technologically for thousands of years.

For most of us here in America and I dare say, around the world, haven't explored world history and ancient civilizations. We have lived in a vacuum more or less that limits our knowledge of what has transpired in the past.

Christian's that limit themselves to just the regions of biblical stories without widening their peripheral knowledge of other civilizations may struggle to grasp the influence of the gods of antiquities. Palms 82

We have show's like Ancient Aliens who has helped open our eyes to some mysteries of the past, but tend to go a step further in assumptions than I would.

Will the world wake up to this reality? That is the question.

Chapter 19

Wake-up Call

The question that we face is, how do we wake people up to the dangers of the strange and often unseen reality of what the human race faces?

I understand people are tired of hearing about Covid. They just want to move on to some normalcy. But if people don't recognize or identify what is taking place, they will continue to leave themselves vulnerable to the deception that was played out upon the world.

It's been a monumental task to wake people up to the reality that our government, the WHO, CDC, NIH and our mainstream media lied to the American public about Covid. Some still believe the government, no matter what evidence is given to counter their claims.

It is about the influence that our government has on people and what they told you to believe.

What was the lie? Only the Covid19 vaccine and boosters could protect you. According to them, there were no treatments or preventive care. However there were in fact treatment and preventative measures for the Covid19 all along.

In order for the government to distribute the dangerous Covid19 vaccine that could not pass standard testing protocols for vaccines, they had to lie to the public about there being no treatment and that the vaccines had a 95 percent efficacy. So they lied to the public about, Ivermectin and Hydroxychloroquine or any other method of treatment. The entire thing was spear headed by the Department of Defense through private companies.

A large part of our public still doesn't know that the so-called vaccine never stopped anyone from getting Covid. It's a blindness that is very difficult to overcome.

So when people hear about invisible entities influencing the elites of our world and heads of states or even UFO's, they shrug it off as though it's not real or just a conspiracy theory.

There will always be those who will scoff and make light of something they have little to no knowledge of. Or they're simply afraid to open their eyes to something that might frighten them or go against their established beliefs.

Back in the 1800s they were saying if man were meant to fly he would have wings. Man will never fly.

Some were saying that we'll never get a vehicle to go over 100 mile per-hour. Just not possible.

Even Einstein theory of relativity was rejected early on by the science community. It took some scientists willing to be neutral and to examine it before it became accepted.

We've all fallen for deception in our lives to one degree or another.

And that is the point. To be willing to hear and willing to see what is transpiring before us. This is a spiritual battle and those who are willing to hear will begin to recognize the influence. But there will always be those who simply can't see and refuse to listen.

Acts 28:27

"For the hearts of these people are hardened,
and their ears cannot hear,
and they have closed their eyes—
so their eyes cannot see,
and their ears cannot hear,
and their hearts cannot understand,
and they cannot turn to me
and let me heal them."

This is what this book is about. The invisible influence that we all face. To recognize that our world leaders are being influenced by these non-human entities that many call fallen angels.

At this writing we are heading into uncharted territory. If former president Donald J. Trump is reelected there is a very strong possibility of riots and turmoil never seen in our last two centuries.

If there are riots as a results of Trump being re-elected, it will be by those who want to destroy our system of government, while claiming they are trying to save democracy.

They must not allow Trump to get back in because he is against globalism: "World Economic Forum (WEF) contributor and Sapiens author Yuval Noah Harari recently said a second Trump term would be **the "death blow" to the global order**."

"Harari implied that Americans' fear of a transition to <u>world government,</u> (he means a one world government) which pushed them to support Trump, is foolish nonsense."

What Harari means by a world government will mean the elimination of what it means to be America.

How the enemy works is through perception. They claim they are trying to help, while doing just the opposite. It's like a murder holding someone's head under the water, and telling on lookers, he is trying to save them.

On top of that, many Americans are still in the dark concerning the possible loss of our sovereignty simply because they have relied upon mainstream news to keep them informed about events in our world. It helps in directing the voting patterns. Not realizing they are keeping them in the dark about our very takeover of our nation.

What our world is about to head into is what some call a soft "Coup-d'etat" or simply, a Coup. It is to bring about a whole new set of laws and to eliminate the existing set laws with nation states. This is what the WEF and the WHO is about.

They hope to bring a global control under the pretext of pandemic awareness or preparedness and a bio-security agenda.

This is being developed through all participating nations with the United States spearheading these treaties.

They're working to place amendments to the existing laws that will replace human rights protections under the IHR's.

Through this they will work to enforce surveillance, censorship and to eliminate freedom of speech as was done during the Covid19 pandemic.

They are pushing the program of vaccines that they will try and have ready for new viruses, (like diseaseX and new emerging viruses) within 100 days that will become mandatory. Doing this through the organization call CEPI.

CEPI stands for, Coalition for Epidemic Preparedness Innovations. One of the supporter's for this organization is the depopulationist, Bill Gates.

<u>CEPI | New Vaccines For A Safer World</u>

This control will all be through the WHO guided by the WEF and United Nations as to help enforce these conditions.

It has been thousands of years of invisible non-human influence that has brought us to the point we are right now.

The invisible influence through the spark of ideas, thought, visions and downloads, where mankind takes them like a runner handing off a baton in a relay race and his knowledge increases.

It was inevitable that man would grow in knowledge.

Dan 12:4

"But you, Daniel, keep these words secret, and seal the book until the end times. Many will travel here and there, and knowledge will grow."

For the last days it was predicted that man would have the capability to travel in ways never before imagined. That his knowledge would increase.

Chapter 20

Unseen Hope

Rom 8:24

"Hope that is seen is not hope. For who hopes for what he sees?"

As of this writing our world and our way of life is at a cross-road. We, as a nation, face many obstacles like: wars, droughts, possible food shortages, political turmoil's that may result in riots, changing values and identities where we can no-longer call a person male or female, staggering looming national debt, crypto or digital currency where every transaction you make will be recorded. Millions of illegals flooding our nation where our leaders force tax payers to pay for their healthcare and education, while our own citizens struggle. Potential dangers from those crossing illegally of terrorist cells and gang members and even talk of Civil War. And on top of all that, our CDC and the WHO are telling the world, we are still in a "pandemic and more is yet to come."

If there ever was a scripture that applies to the word "hope," it's Romans 8:24. Because people are hoping that we will find ways to survive and come through this present time of trouble.

We are "hoping" right now, that we'll find a way through what we as nation and the world, face. But we physically don't see the solution right now. So we HOPE.

Let me point out. When Romans 8:24 talks about hope. The writer was actually talking about the salvation of our body through Jesus Christ.

The writer, believed to be the Apostle Paul, talked about the creation being in pain like that of birthing a child and that someday, like our body, creation will put off that part where it decays. But that hasn't happened yet, and so we hope.

In like manor, the solution to our deteriorating culture and way of life brings us to the point of, hope. We hope we can come through this time of trouble and find peace and rest.

You may have heard people say, I can't even watch the news any longer, it's too depressing. People just want peace and rest for their souls.

The reality is, in this world there's always going to be unrest and trouble. Yes there will be times of ease for those of us who have the means to live in comfort and avoid the looming trouble, but only for a time.

This is what many don't realize. Whether you're a Christian believer or not, the person Jesus, who is also a dimensional being, is God's only son. In other words, Jesus is the only one that has the same nature of God the father, who created all things through the son.

This is why Jesus said in John 14:8-9:

"Philip said to him, "Lord, show us the Father, and it is enough for us." 9 Jesus said to him, "Have I been with you so long, and you still do not know me, Philip? Whoever has seen me has seen the Father." ESV

Everyone wants to find peace and rest that is everlasting. However for those who are willing to listen, it is Jesus telling us how that happens: Matt 11:28-30

28 Come to me, all who labor and are heavy laden, and I will give you rest. 29 Take my yoke upon you, and learn from me, for I am gentle and lowly in heart, and you will find rest for your souls. 30 For my yoke is easy, and my burden is light." ESV

John 16:33

3 I have told you all this so that you may have peace in me. Here on earth you will have many trials and sorrows. But take heart, because I have overcome the world."

In other words, Jesus, who created all things, is offering those of us who are willing to listen and believe on him, that we can find that internal peace though him; even in the middle of troublesome times.

He's not saying you'll be void of pain and sorrow. It's a peace that isn't found in the things of the world. It's a peace of knowing that he offers life beyond this world.

It is that internal peace that he offers knowing life on this planet will not allow anyone to escape trials and sorrows. But that internal peace can be found in him, Jesus.

Jesus provided us, who are willing to listen and believe, an eventual escape from this life here that brings trials and sorrows.

John 3:16-17

6 For God so loved the world that He gave His only begotten Son, that whoever believes in Him should not perish but have everlasting life. 17 For God did not send His Son into the world to condemn the world, but that the world through Him might be saved. NKJV

Conflict and trouble will be a part of this physical life we have here. But through it all, we can still find a peace and rest within us through Jesus Christ.

We face an invisible foe and the battleground that takes place is within our minds. We struggle by what we see coming and worry. That is natural for all us. Yet this person called Jesus, and who is the creator of our world and time and space, offers us the way to find that peace.

Because the failures that we've had in this life, Jesus stepped up and paid the price for our failures and wipes them clean and all it takes is that first step in believing on him.

Rom 10:9-11

9 If you confess with your mouth that Jesus is Lord and believe in your heart that God raised him from the dead, you will be saved. 10 For it is by believing in your heart that you are made right with God, and it is by confessing with your mouth that you are saved.

We are in a historical battle that started with the creation of man.

The invisible entities, some call alien and others call fallen angels or demons, have influenced mankind and the elites throughout history. It reveals that these entities deceive and use man's nature as a catalyst to bring strife and turmoil and man, apart from God, will fall prey to the influence of these entities.

Rev 12:7-10:

7 Then there was war in heaven. Michael and his angels fought against the dragon and his angels. 8 And the dragon lost the battle, and he and his angels

were forced out of heaven. 9 This great dragon—the ancient serpent called the devil, or Satan, <u>the one deceiving the whole world</u>—was thrown down to the earth with all his angels.

10 Then I heard a loud voice shouting across the heavens,
"It has come at last—
salvation and power
and the Kingdom of our God,
and the authority of his Christ.

That authority was given to Christ when he was raised from the dead after being crucified.

Matt 28:17-18:

17 And when they saw him, they worshipped him: but some doubted.

18 And Jesus came and spoke to them, saying, All power is given unto me in heaven and in earth. KJV

The age old battle from the birth of the human race is, good vs evil. Within this historical battle God offers mankind an eternal peace not found in the things of this world.

We know that we all must face what comes our way. We know those leading nations and those at the very seat of power tend to eventually bring hardship and sorry over those they rule.

So how do we find that inner peace during the hardships and sorrow?

Jesus said this:

John 10:10

"The thief comes only to steal and kill and destroy. I came that they may have life and have it abundantly." ESV

For the Christian believer, you must understand, that when Jesus uses the word abundantly, he wasn't referring to you getting rich or having more material things.

Being rich or having material things isn't a sin. Only if that consumes your life does it then become a chain around a person's neck.

Jesus spoke in parables. The word "abundantly" in the Greek is "perisson" and means: superior, extraordinary, surpassing, uncommon.

What Jesus was saying, while the enemy may bring pain, sorrow and hardship, the peace that he gives will be uncommon, surpassing the natural peace found in this world.

Epilogue

Mankind along with the rulers and elites of our world throughout history have been manipulated and used like chest pieces in strategic maneuvers.

Entities have used mankind to create wars, conflicts and divisions throughout would history.

It is a war set in motion from the very beginning. The very reality of what exists in our world and even among us have been cloaked through unbelief by the masses. Even those who are Christian fail to recognize the invisible influence that plagues our world today.

The blinders are slowly being removed. For years everyone believed UFO's were just the imagination of unstable people. That is what part of our government, with the help of mainstream media, manipulated the public to believe.

Along with pulling back these blinders on UFO or UAPs, will be the revelation that the UFO is only a small part of what really is taking place.

There are dimensional entities that have been here from the very beginning of mankind. These entities are in fact a creation of God that rebelled. They can take many different forms for the purpose of deceiving man and those they contact.

So what is the hope for America?

We all want to believe and have faith that America will pull through and that virtue, honor and character will win out.

Will that happen? I don't know. The only thing I know is whether you are a person of faith or a person of high moral values, we all must fight for what we know to be right.

For people of faith, our true hope is not found in America but in Christ who was willing to pay the price for our failures. Christ is our perpetuation

Heb 9:15

Through his death he paid the price to set people free from the sins they committed under the first promise. He did this so that those who are called can be guaranteed an inheritance that will last forever.

The likelihood is very few will read this book. But those who have taken the time to read through it, will now be armed with the knowledge that there's an invisible enemy manipulating events in our world through the elites.

The battleground is your mind and Christ is our safe haven.

www.ingramcontent.com/pod-product-compliance
Lightning Source LLC
Chambersburg PA
CBHW052254220526
45471CB00001B/325